5.50

EIGHTH EDITION

AF768892

Supplement to

Handbook on Injectable Drugs

by Lawrence A. Trissel

ASHP®

LAWRENCE A. TRISSEL, FASHP, the author of the *Handbook on Injectable Drugs*, is Director, Drug Delivery and Stability Research, Division of Pharmacy, University of Texas, M. D. Anderson Cancer Center, Houston.

Mr. Trissel was assisted in the preparation of this Supplement by KAREN NAQUIN HALE, Clinical Specialist, Investigational Drug Service, Department of Pharmacy, The Ohio State University Medical Center, and Clinical Assistant Professor, The Ohio State University College of Pharmacy.

Correspondence to the author should be sent in care of the publisher, American Society of Health-System Pharmacists, 7272 Wisconsin Avenue, Bethesda, MD 20814.

The information presented herein reflects the opinions of the author(s) and reviewer(s). It should not be interpreted as official policy of ASHP or as an endorsement of any product(s).

Drug information is constantly evolving because of ongoing research and clinical experience, and it is often subject to interpretation and the uniqueness of a clinical situation. The author and ASHP have made every effort to ensure the accuracy and completeness of the information presented in this book. However, the reader is advised that the publisher, author, contributors, editors, and reviewers cannot be responsible for the continued currency of the information, for any errors or omissions, and for any consequences arising therefrom.

Produced by the American Society of Health-System Pharmacists' Special Projects Division.

Cover design: Hector L. Coronado

©1995, American Society of Health-System Pharmacists, Inc. All rights reserved.

No part of this publication may be reproduced or transmitted in any form or by any means, electronic or mechanical, including photocopying, microfilming, and recording, or by any information storage and retrieval system, without written permission from the American Society of Health-System Pharmacists.

ASHP® is a service mark of the American Society of Health-System Pharmacists, Inc.; registered in the U.S. Patent and Trademark Office.

ISBN: 1-879907-54-2

TABLE OF CONTENTS

Preface iv

New Commercial Drug Monographs 1
  Flumazenil 3
  Sufentanil Citrate 4
  Tacrolimus 5
  Vinorelbine Tartrate 8

Additions to Commercial Drug Monograph Tables 19

Appendix I: Parenteral Nutrition Solution Formulas 87

References 89

PREFACE

This Supplement contains information from published articles that were obtained following data input to the eighth edition of the *Handbook on Injectable Drugs*. This Supplement primarily consists of new entries into the compatibility tables of existing monographs in the *Handbook.* However, four new monographs appear in the first section:

Flumazenil
Sufentanil citrate
Tacrolimus
Vinorelbine tartrate

As in the *Handbook*, the information is arranged alphabetically by nonproprietary name. The *American Hospital Formulary Service* category number and the citation to the original *Handbook* monograph are included to aid the user. The new table inserts are cited under the familiar table headings for solution, additive, drugs in syringe, and Y-site injection compatibility.

Appendix I contains additional formulas for parenteral nutrition solutions. New references appear at the end of this Supplement.

For a complete description of the monograph and table formats, refer to the How to Use the Handbook section, pages IX–XII, in the eighth edition.

For easy access to the new information, keep this Supplement with your *Handbook on Injectable Drugs*. The Supplement should be used until the next edition of the *Handbook* is published. The new edition will incorporate the Supplement information plus all data appearing after its preparation.

Additions to Manufacturer and Compendium Abbreviations
(*Handbook on Injectable Drugs*, eighth edition, page XII)

GRU	Grunenthal
MAR	Marsam
TAK	Takeda

Correction to Eighth Edition
TRIMETHOPRIM–SULFAMETHOXAZOLE
On page 1023 under *Syringes,* the first sentence should read:

> "Undiluted trimethoprim–sulfamethoxazole (Elkins-Sinn) (16 + 80 mg/ml) was stored in polypropylene syringes (Becton-Dickinson) for two and a half days at room temperature."

LAT
April 1995

New Commercial Drug Monographs

FLUMAZENIL
AHFS 92:00

Romazicon **Roche**

Products— Flumazenil (Roche) is available as a 0.1-mg/ml solution in 5- and 10-ml multiple-dose vials. In addition to flumazenil, each milliliter also contains methylparaben 1.8 mg, propylparaben 0.2 mg, sodium chloride 0.9%, edetate disodium 0.01%, and acetic acid 0.01%. The pH is adjusted with hydrochloric acid and, if necessary, sodium hydroxide (1-4/93).

pH— The injection has a pH of approximately 4 (1-4/93).

Dosage— Flumazenil is administered intravenously either directly or diluted in a compatible infusion solution. To minimize pain at the injection site, flumazenil should be administered through a freely running intravenous infusion line into a large vein. The administration should not be rushed (1-4/93).

The dose of flumazenil should be individualized to the patient's need and response. For reversal of conscious sedation or in general anesthesia, the usual initial dose is 0.2 mg administered over 15 seconds. If the desired level of consciousness is not obtained after 45 seconds, an additional 0.2 mg can be injected. If needed, an additional 0.2 mg then can be injected at 60-second intervals for up to four additional doses, with a maximum total dose of 1 mg (1-4/93).

In the event of resedation, repeat doses may be given at 20-minute intervals. No more than 1 mg should be given at one time, nor should more than 3 mg be given in one hour (1-4/93).

For suspected benzodiazepine overdose, the usual initial dose is 0.2 mg intravenously over 30 seconds. If the desired level of consciousness is not obtained after 30 seconds, a dose of 0.3 mg can be administered over 30 seconds. If needed, additional 0.5-mg doses can be given over 30 to 60 seconds, with a maximum total dose of 5 mg (1-4/93).

Stability— Flumazenil injection (Roche) is a stable aqueous solution; it should be stored at controlled room temperature (15 to 30 °C). The manufacturer recommends discarding the product 24 hours after removal from its original vial, whether admixed in an infusion solution or simply drawn into a syringe (1-4/93).

Compatibility Information

Solution Compatibility

Flumazenil

Solution	*Mfr*	*Mfr*	*Conc/L*	*Remarks*	*Ref*	*C/I*
Dextrose 5% in water	BA[a]	RC	20 mg	Visually compatible with no flumazenil loss by HPLC in 24 hr at 23 °C under fluorescent light	1710	C

[a]*Tested in PVC containers.*

Additive Compatibility

Flumazenil

Drug	*Mfr*	*Conc/L*	*Mfr*	*Conc/L*	*Test Soln*	*Remarks*	*Ref*	*C/I*
Aminophylline	AMR	2 g	RC	20 mg	D5W[a]	Visually compatible with no flumazenil loss by HPLC in 24 hr at 23 °C under fluorescent light. Aminophylline not tested	1710	C
Cimetidine HCl	SKB	2.4 g	RC	20 mg	D5W[a]	Visually compatible with no flumazenil loss by HPLC in 24 hr at 23 °C under fluorescent light. Cimetidine not tested	1710	C
Dobutamine HCl	LI	2 g	RC	20 mg	D5W[a]	Visually compatible with no flumazenil loss by HPLC in 24 hr at 23 °C under fluorescent light. Dobutamine not tested	1710	C
Dopamine HCl	AB	3.2 g	RC	20 mg	D5W[a]	Visually compatible with 7% flumazenil loss by HPLC in 24 hr at 23 °C under fluorescent light. Dopamine not tested	1710	C
Famotidine	MSD	80 mg	RC	20 mg	D5W[a]	Visually compatible with 3% flumazenil loss by HPLC in 24 hr at 23 °C under fluorescent light. Famotidine not tested	1710	C
Heparin sodium	ES	50,000 units	RC	20 mg	D5W[a]	Visually compatible with 4% flumazenil loss by HPLC in 24 hr at 23 °C under fluorescent light. Heparin not tested	1710	C

Additive Compatibility (Cont.)

Flumazenil

Drug	*Mfr*	*Conc/L*	*Mfr*	*Conc/L*	*Test Soln*	*Remarks*	*Ref*	*C/I*
Lidocaine HCl	AB	4 g	RC	20 mg	D5W[a]	Visually compatible with 4% flumazenil loss by HPLC in 24 hr at 23 °C under fluorescent light. Lidocaine not tested	1710	**C**
Procainamide HCl	ES	4 g	RC	20 mg	D5W[a]	Visually compatible with no flumazenil loss by HPLC in 24 hr at 23 °C under fluorescent light. Procainamide not tested	1710	**C**
Ranitidine HCl	GL	300 mg	RC	20 mg	D5W[a]	Visually compatible with 3% flumazenil loss by HPLC in 24 hr at 23 °C under fluorescent light. Ranitidine not tested	1710	**C**

[a]*Tested in PVC containers.*

Additional Compatibility Information

Solutions— The manufacturer states that flumazenil is compatible with dextrose 5% in water, sodium chloride 0.9%, and Ringer's injection, lactated (1-4/93).

SUFENTANIL CITRATE
AHFS 28:08.08

Sufenta **Janssen**

Products— Sufentanil citrate (Janssen) is available as a preservative-free aqueous injection in 1-, 2-, and 5-ml ampuls. Each milliliter of solution contains sufentanil citrate equivalent to 50 μg of sufentanil base (1-11/93).

pH— From 3.5 to 6 (1-11/93).

Dosage— Sufentanil citrate is administered intravenously by slow injection or infusion. For labor and delivery, it may be administered epidurally (1-11/93; 4). The drug has also been administered intramuscularly (4).

Dosage should be individualized for each patient's needs and response. The total intravenous analgesic dose usually is 1 to 2 μg/kg for anesthesia of one to two hours or 2 to 8 μg/kg for anesthesia of two to eight hours. Incremental doses of 10 to 50 μg may be administered when movement and/or changes in vital signs indicate lightening of analgesia (1-11/93; 4).

As an anesthetic, total doses of 8 to 30 μg/kg may be administered as a slow injection, an infusion, or an injection followed by an infusion. Depending on the initial dose, maintenance doses of 0.5 to 10 μg/kg may be administered by slow injection. The drug may also be administered by continuous or intermittent infusion in response to lightening of anesthesia. The maintenance infusion rate should be based on the induction dose so that the total dose does not exceed 30 μg/kg (1-11/93).

Dosage should be reduced in elderly or debilitated patients. Adjustments may also be required in patients with renal or hepatic impairment. Concomitant administration of other CNS depressants may require reduced doses of sufentanil citrate and/or the other drugs (1-11/93; 4).

For epidural use in labor and delivery, the recommended dose of sufentanil citrate is 10 to 15 μg administered with 10 ml of bupivacaine 0.125%, with or without epinephrine. Doses can be repeated twice (three doses total) at intervals of one or more hours until delivery (1-11/93).

In children two to 12 years of age, an anesthetic dose of 10 to 25 μg/kg is recommended. Supplemental doses of 25 to 50 μg (up to a total of 1 to 2 μg/kg) are recommended for maintenance, based on the patient's response and changes in vital signs or lightening of anesthesia (1-11/93; 4). Dosage in children less than two years of age has not been established (4).

Stability— Sufentanil citrate (Janssen) is a stable, clear, aqueous, preservative-free injection. The product should be stored at controlled room temperature (15 to 30 °C) and protected from light (1-11/93; 4). It is hydrolyzed in acidic solutions (4).

Filtration— Sufentanil citrate (Janssen) 50 μg/10 ml in sodium chloride 0.9% was evaluated for drug loss when administered through filters or epidural catheters; 2.5-g cellulose acetate/cellulose nitrate 0.2-μm filters (Millex, Millipore) were utilized. Approximately 20% of the sufentanil was lost to the void volume and/or adsorption. This loss should be considered when a new filter is used (1667).

Compatibility Information

Drugs in Syringe Compatibility

Sufentanil citrate

Drug (in syringe)	*Mfr*	*Amt*	*Mfr*	*Amt*	*Remarks*	*Ref*	*C/I*
Atracurium besylate	BW	10 mg/ml		50 μg/ml	Physically compatible and atracurium chemically stable for 24 hr at 5 and 25 °C	1694	**C**
Atropine sulfate	LY	0.4 mg/ml	JN	50 μg/ml	Physically compatible with no change in measured turbidity or increase in particle content in 24 hr at 23 °C under fluorescent light	1711	**C**
Dexamethasone sodium phosphate	AMR	4 mg/ml	JN	50 μg/ml	Physically compatible with no change in measured turbidity or increase in particle content in 24 hr at 23 °C under fluorescent light	1711	**C**
Diazepam	ES	5 mg/ml	JN	50 μg/ml	White turbidity forms immediately. Precipitate forms in 24 hr at 23 °C	1711	**I**
Diphenhydramine HCl	SCN	50 mg/ml	JN	50 μg/ml	Physically compatible with no change in measured turbidity or increase in particle content in 24 hr at 23 °C under fluorescent light	1711	**C**
Haloperidol lactate	MN	5 mg/ml	JN	50 μg/ml	Physically compatible with no change in measured turbidity or increase in particle content in 24 hr at 23 °C under fluorescent light	1711	**C**
Hydroxyzine HCl	ES	50 mg/ml	JN	50 μg/ml	Physically compatible with no change in measured turbidity or increase in particle content in 24 hr at 23 °C under fluorescent light	1711	**C**
Ketorolac tromethamine	WY	30 mg/ml	JN	50 μg/ml	Physically compatible with no change in measured turbidity or increase in particle content in 24 hr at 23 °C under fluorescent light	1711	**C**
Lorazepam	WY	2 mg/ml	JN	50 μg/ml	Turbidity increases within 0.5 hr and continues to increase over 24 hr at 23 °C	1711	**I**
Methotrimeprazine	LE	20 mg/ml	JN	50 μg/ml	Physically compatible with no change in measured turbidity or increase in particle content in 24 hr at 23 °C under fluorescent light	1711	**C**
Metoclopramide HCl	RB	5 mg/ml	JN	50 μg/ml	Physically compatible with no change in measured turbidity or increase in particle content in 24 hr at 23 °C under fluorescent light	1711	**C**
Midazolam HCl	RC	5 mg/ml	JN	50 μg/ml	Physically compatible with no change in measured turbidity or increase in particle content in 24 hr at 23 °C under fluorescent light	1711	**C**
Phenobarbital sodium	WY	60 mg/ml	JN	50 μg/ml	Haze forms immediately and particles form in 24 hr at 23 °C	1711	**I**
Phenytoin sodium	SO	50 mg/ml	JN	50 μg/ml	Small crystals form immediately. Large crystals settle to bottom in 24 hr at 23 °C	1711	**I**

Drugs in Syringe Compatibility (Cont.)

Sufentanil citrate

Drug (in syringe)	*Mfr*	*Amt*	*Mfr*	*Amt*	*Remarks*	*Ref*	*C/I*
Prochlorperazine edisylate	SCN	5 mg/ml	JN	50 μg/ml	Physically compatible with no change in measured turbidity or increase in particle content in 24 hr at 23 °C under fluorescent light	1711	C
Scopolamine HBr	LY	0.43 mg/ml	JN	50 μg/ml	Physically compatible with no change in measured turbidity or increase in particle content in 24 hr at 23 °C under fluorescent light	1711	C

Y-Site Injection Compatibility (1:1 Mixture)

Sufentanil citrate

Drug	*Mfr*	*Conc*	*Mfr*	*Conc*	*Remarks*	*Ref*	*C/I*
Atropine sulfate	LY	0.4 mg/ml[a]	JN	12.5 μg/ml[a]	Physically compatible with no change in measured turbidity or increase in particle content in 24 hr at 23 °C under fluorescent light	1711	C
Dexamethasone sodium phosphate	AMR	1 mg/ml[a]	JN	12.5 μg/ml[a]	Physically compatible with no change in measured turbidity or increase in particle content in 24 hr at 23 °C under fluorescent light	1711	C
Diazepam	ES	0.5 mg/ml[a]	JN	12.5 μg/ml[a]	Physically compatible with no change in measured turbidity or increase in particle content in 24 hr at 23 °C under fluorescent light	1711	C
Diphenhydramine HCl	SCN	2 mg/ml[a]	JN	12.5 μg/ml[a]	Physically compatible with no change in measured turbidity or increase in particle content in 24 hr at 23 °C under fluorescent light	1711	C
Haloperidol lactate	MN	0.2 mg/ml[a]	JN	12.5 μg/ml[a]	Physically compatible with no change in measured turbidity or increase in particle content in 24 hr at 23 °C under fluorescent light	1711	C
Hydroxyzine HCl	ES	4 mg/ml[a]	JN	12.5 μg/ml[a]	Physically compatible with little change in measured turbidity or increase in particle content in 24 hr at 23 °C under fluorescent light	1711	C
Ketorolac tromethamine	SY	1 mg/ml[a]	JN	12.5 μg/ml[a]	Physically compatible with no change in measured turbidity or increase in particle content in 24 hr at 23 °C under fluorescent light	1711	C
Lorazepam	WY	0.1 mg/ml[a]	JN	12.5 μg/ml[a]	Large increase in measured turbidity occurs immediately and persists for 24 hr at 23 °C under fluorescent light	1711	I
Methotrimeprazine	LE	0.2 mg/ml[a]	JN	12.5 μg/ml[a]	Physically compatible with no change in measured turbidity or increase in particle content in 24 hr at 23 °C under fluorescent light	1711	C

Y-Site Injection Compatibility (1:1 Mixture) (Cont.)

Sufentanil citrate

Drug	*Mfr*	*Conc*	*Mfr*	*Conc*	*Remarks*	*Ref*	*C/I*
Metoclopramide HCl	RB	5 mg/ml	JN	12.5 μg/ml[a]	Physically compatible with no change in measured turbidity or increase in particle content in 24 hr at 23 °C under fluorescent light	1711	C
Midazolam HCl	RC	0.2 mg/ml[a]	JN	12.5 μg/ml[a]	Physically compatible with no change in measured turbidity or increase in particle content in 24 hr at 23 °C under fluorescent light	1711	C
Phenobarbital sodium	WY	2 mg/ml[a]	JN	12.5 μg/ml[a]	Physically compatible with no change in measured turbidity or increase in particle content in 24 hr at 23 °C under fluorescent light	1711	C
Phenytoin sodium	ES	2 mg/ml[a]	JN	12.5 μg/ml[a]	Numerous tiny crystals form immediately and become larger over 24 hr at 23 °C under fluorescent light	1711	I
Prochlorperazine edisylate	SCN	0.5 mg/ml[a]	JN	12.5 μg/ml[a]	Physically compatible with little change in measured turbidity or increase in particle content in 24 hr at 23 °C under fluorescent light	1711	C
Scopolamine HBr	LY	0.05 mg/ml[a]	JN	12.5 μg/ml[a]	Physically compatible with no change in measured turbidity or increase in particle content in 24 hr at 23 °C under fluorescent light	1711	C

[a]Tested in dextrose 5% in water.

TACROLIMUS
AHFS 92:00

Prograf **Fujisawa**

Products— Tacrolimus injection (Fujisawa) is available in 1-ml ampuls containing the equivalent of 5 mg of anhydrous tacrolimus per milliliter. In addition to tacrolimus, each milliliter contains polyoxyl 60 hydrogenated castor oil (surfactant) 200 mg and dehydrated alcohol, USP, 80% (v/v). The product is a concentrate that must be diluted for use (1-4/94).

Dosage— Tacrolimus is administered by intravenous infusion. The drug must be diluted to a final concentration of 0.004 to 0.02 mg/ml in dextrose 5% in water or sodium chloride 0.9%. Intravenous solution containers should be made of glass or polyethylene; PVC containers plasticized with diethylhexyl phthalate (DEHP) should be avoided due to leaching of plasticizer and decreased stability (1-4/94). Similarly, a non-DEHP plasticized administration set should be used to avoid plasticizer leaching.

The initial dose is administered no sooner than six hours after transplantation. The starting dose is 0.05 to 0.1 mg/kg/day as a continuous intravenous infusion. Adults should receive doses at the lower end of the range. Pediatric patients without preexisting renal or hepatic dysfunction should be started at the high end (0.1 mg/kg/day) (1-4/94).

Patients with renal or hepatic impairment should receive the lowest recommended doses, and further reductions may be necessary (1-4/94).

Compatibility Information

Y-Site Injection Compatibility (1:1 Mixture)

Tacrolimus

Drug	*Mfr*	*Conc*	*Mfr*	*Conc*	*Remarks*	*Ref*	*C/I*
Acyclovir sodium	BW	10 mg/ml[a]	FUJ	1 mg/ml[b]	Visually compatible for 24 hr at 25 °C under fluorescent light	1630	C

Tacrolimus

Drug	*Mfr*	*Conc*	*Mfr*	*Conc*	*Remarks*	*Ref*	*C/I*
Aminophylline	ES	2 mg/ml[a]	FUJ	1 mg/ml[b]	Visually compatible for 24 hr at 25 °C under fluorescent light	1630	**C**
Amphotericin B	LY	5 mg/ml[a]	FUJ	1 mg/ml[c]	Visually compatible for 24 hr at 25 °C under fluorescent light	1630	**C**
Ampicillin sodium	WY	20 mg/ml[a]	FUJ	1 mg/ml[b]	Visually compatible for 24 hr at 25 °C under fluorescent light	1630	**C**
Ampicillin sodium–sulbactam sodium	RR	50 mg/ml[a]	FUJ	1 mg/ml[b]	Visually compatible for 24 hr at 25 °C under fluorescent light	1630	**C**
Benztropine mesylate	MSD	1 mg/ml[a]	FUJ	1 mg/ml[b]	Visually compatible for 24 hr at 25 °C under fluorescent light	1630	**C**
Calcium gluconate	ES	100 mg/ml	FUJ	1 mg/ml[b]	Visually compatible for 24 hr at 25 °C under fluorescent light	1630	**C**
Cefazolin sodium	BR	40 mg/ml[a]	FUJ	1 mg/ml[b]	Visually compatible for 24 hr at 25 °C under fluorescent light	1630	**C**
Cefotetan disodium	STU	40 mg/ml[a]	FUJ	1 mg/ml[b]	Visually compatible for 24 hr at 25 °C under fluorescent light	1630	**C**
Ceftazidime	GL	20 mg/ml[a]	FUJ	1 mg/ml[b]	Visually compatible for 24 hr at 25 °C under fluorescent light	1630	**C**
Ceftriaxone sodium	RC	40 mg/ml[a]	FUJ	1 mg/ml[b]	Visually compatible for 24 hr at 25 °C under fluorescent light	1630	**C**
Cefuroxime sodium	LI	30 mg/ml[a]	FUJ	1 mg/ml[b]	Visually compatible for 24 hr at 25 °C under fluorescent light	1630	**C**
Chloramphenicol sodium succinate	PD	20 mg/ml[a]	FUJ	1 mg/ml[b]	Visually compatible for 24 hr at 25 °C under fluorescent light	1630	**C**
Cimetidine HCl	SKB	150 mg/ml[a]	FUJ	1 mg/ml[b]	Visually compatible for 24 hr at 25 °C under fluorescent light	1630	**C**
Ciprofloxacin	MI	1 mg/ml[a]	FUJ	1 mg/ml[b]	Visually compatible for 24 hr at 25 °C under fluorescent light	1630	**C**
Clindamycin phosphate	ES	12 mg/ml[a]	FUJ	1 mg/ml[b]	Visually compatible for 24 hr at 25 °C under fluorescent light	1630	**C**
Dexamethasone sodium phosphate	ES	4 mg/ml[a]	FUJ	1 mg/ml[b]	Visually compatible for 24 hr at 25 °C under fluorescent light	1630	**C**
Digoxin	WY	0.25 mg/ml	FUJ	1 mg/ml[b]	Visually compatible for 24 hr at 25 °C under fluorescent light	1630	**C**
Diphenhydramine HCl	ES	1 mg/ml[a]	FUJ	1 mg/ml[b]	Visually compatible for 24 hr at 25 °C under fluorescent light	1630	**C**
Dobutamine HCl	LI	1 mg/ml[a]	FUJ	1 mg/ml[b]	Visually compatible for 24 hr at 25 °C under fluorescent light	1630	**C**
Dopamine HCl	ES	1.6 mg/ml[a]	FUJ	1 mg/ml[b]	Visually compatible for 24 hr at 25 °C under fluorescent light	1630	**C**
Doxycycline hyclate	RR	5 mg/ml[a]	FUJ	1 mg/ml[b]	Visually compatible for 24 hr at 25 °C under fluorescent light	1630	**C**
Erythromycin lactobionate	AB	20 mg/ml[a]	FUJ	1 mg/ml[b]	Visually compatible for 24 hr at 25 °C under fluorescent light	1630	**C**
Esmolol HCl	DU	10 mg/ml[a]	FUJ	1 mg/ml[b]	Visually compatible for 24 hr at 25 °C under fluorescent light	1630	**C**

Tacrolimus

Drug	*Mfr*	*Conc*	*Mfr*	*Conc*	*Remarks*	*Ref*	*C/I*
Fluconazole	RR	2 mg/ml[a]	FUJ	1 mg/ml[b]	Visually compatible for 24 hr at 25 °C under fluorescent light	1630	C
Furosemide	ES	10 mg/ml	FUJ	1 mg/ml[b]	Visually compatible for 24 hr at 25 °C under fluorescent light	1630	C
Ganciclovir sodium	SY	50 mg/ml[a]	FUJ	1 mg/ml[b]	Visually compatible for 24 hr at 25 °C under fluorescent light	1630	C
Gentamicin sulfate	SCN	4 mg/ml[a]	FUJ	1 mg/ml[b]	Visually compatible for 24 hr at 25 °C under fluorescent light	1630	C
Haloperidol lactate	SO	2.5 mg/ml[a]	FUJ	1 mg/ml[b]	Visually compatible for 24 hr at 25 °C under fluorescent light	1630	C
Heparin sodium	ES	10 units/ml[a]	FUJ	1 mg/ml[b]	Visually compatible for 24 hr at 25 °C under fluorescent light	1630	C
Hydrocortisone sodium succinate	AB	50 mg/ml[a]	FUJ	1 mg/ml[b]	Visually compatible for 24 hr at 25 °C under fluorescent light	1630	C
Imipenem–cilastatin sodium	MSD	10 mg/ml[b]	FUJ	1 mg/ml[b]	Visually compatible for 24 hr at 25 °C under fluorescent light	1630	C
Insulin, regular	LI	0.1 unit/ml[a]	FUJ	1 mg/ml[b]	Visually compatible for 24 hr at 25 °C under fluorescent light	1630	C
Isoproterenol HCl	ES	0.04 mg/ml[a]	FUJ	1 mg/ml[b]	Visually compatible for 24 hr at 25 °C under fluorescent light	1630	C
Leucovorin calcium	ES	10 mg/ml[a]	FUJ	1 mg/ml[b]	Visually compatible for 24 hr at 25 °C under fluorescent light	1630	C
Lorazepam	WY	1 mg/ml[a]	FUJ	1 mg/ml[b]	Visually compatible for 24 hr at 25 °C under fluorescent light	1630	C
Methylprednisolone sodium succinate	UP	0.8 mg/ml[a]	FUJ	1 mg/ml[b]	Visually compatible for 24 hr at 25 °C under fluorescent light	1630	C
Metoclopramide HCl	DU	0.2 mg/ml[a]	FUJ	1 mg/ml[b]	Visually compatible for 24 hr at 25 °C under fluorescent light	1630	C
Metronidazole	AB	5 mg/ml[a]	FUJ	1 mg/ml[b]	Visually compatible for 24 hr at 25 °C under fluorescent light	1630	C
Mezlocillin sodium	MI	40 mg/ml[a]	FUJ	1 mg/ml[b]	Visually compatible for 24 hr at 25 °C under fluorescent light	1630	C
Multivitamins	LY	0.001 ml/ml[a]	FUJ	1 mg/ml[b]	Visually compatible for 24 hr at 25 °C under fluorescent light	1630	C
Nitroglycerin	DU	0.1 mg/ml[a]	FUJ	1 mg/ml[b]	Visually compatible for 24 hr at 25 °C under fluorescent light	1630	C
Oxacillin sodium	BR	40 mg/ml[a]	FUJ	1 mg/ml[b]	Visually compatible for 24 hr at 25 °C under fluorescent light	1630	C
Penicillin G potassium	BR	100,000 units/ml[a]	FUJ	1 mg/ml[b]	Visually compatible for 24 hr at 25 °C under fluorescent light	1630	C
Perphenazine	SC	2.5 mg/ml[a]	FUJ	1 mg/ml[b]	Visually compatible for 24 hr at 25 °C under fluorescent light	1630	C
Phenytoin sodium	ES	5 mg/ml[a]	FUJ	1 mg/ml[b]	Visually compatible for 4 hr at 25 °C under fluorescent light. White haze forms by 24 hr	1630	C

Tacrolimus

Drug	*Mfr*	*Conc*	*Mfr*	*Conc*	*Remarks*	*Ref*	*C/I*
Piperacillin sodium	LE	80 mg/ml[a]	FUJ	1 mg/ml[b]	Visually compatible for 24 hr at 25 °C under fluorescent light	1630	C
Potassium chloride	AB	2 mEq/ml	FUJ	1 mg/ml[b]	Visually compatible for 24 hr at 25 °C under fluorescent light	1630	C
Propranolol HCl	AY	1 mg/ml	FUJ	1 mg/ml[b]	Visually compatible for 24 hr at 25 °C under fluorescent light	1630	C
Ranitidine HCl	GL	25 mg/ml[a]	FUJ	1 mg/ml[b]	Visually compatible for 24 hr at 25 °C under fluorescent light	1630	C
Sodium bicarbonate	AB	1 mEq/ml	FUJ	1 mg/ml[b]	Visually compatible for 24 hr at 25 °C under fluorescent light	1630	C
Sodium nitroprusside	ES	0.004 mg/ml[a]	FUJ	1 mg/ml[b]	Visually compatible for 24 hr at 25 °C under fluorescent light	1630	C
Sodium tetradecyl sulfate	ES	10 mg/ml	FUJ	1 mg/ml[b]	Visually compatible for 24 hr at 25 °C under fluorescent light	1630	C
Tobramycin sulfate	BR	40 mg/ml	FUJ	1 mg/ml[b]	Visually compatible for 24 hr at 25 °C under fluorescent light	1630	C
Trimethoprim–sulfamethoxazole	RC	1.6 + 8 mg/ml[a]	FUJ	1 mg/ml[b]	Visually compatible for 24 hr at 25 °C under fluorescent light	1630	C
Vancomycin HCl	LI	5 mg/ml[a]	FUJ	1 mg/ml[b]	Visually compatible for 24 hr at 25 °C under fluorescent light	1630	C

[a]*Tested in dextrose 5% in water.*
[b]*Tested in sodium chloride 0.9%.*
[c]*Diluted with sterile water for injection.*

Additional Compatibility Information

Solutions— The manufacturer recommends dilution of tacrolimus to 0.004 to 0.02 mg/ml in dextrose 5% in water or sodium chloride 0.9%. These solutions are reported to be stable for 24 hours (1-4/94).

Plasticizer Extraction— Parenteral products containing a large amount of a surfactant will extract the plasticizer DEHP from PVC containers and administration sets. Consequently, their use should be avoided. Instead, glass or polyethylene containers and non-DEHP plasticized administration sets are recommended (1-4/94).

VINORELBINE TARTRATE
AHFS 10:00

Navelbine **Burroughs Wellcome**

Products— Vinorelbine tartrate (Burroughs Wellcome) is available in a 10-mg/ml concentration in water for injection in 1- and 5-ml single-use vials. No preservatives or other additives are present (1-12/94).

Vinorelbine tartrate should be diluted with a compatible diluent for administration. Because skin reactions may occur, gloves should be worn during preparation (1-12/94).

pH— The injection has a pH of approximately 3.5 (1-12/94).

Dosage— Vinorelbine tartrate is administered intravenously, after dilution, from a syringe (at a concentration of 1.5 to 3 mg/ml) or infusion solution minibag (at a concentration of 0.5 to 2 mg/ml) over 6 to 10 minutes into the side port of a free-flowing infusion solution closest to the infusion container. After administration, 75 to 125 ml of solution should be used as a flush. Extravasation should be avoided due to tissue irritation, necrosis, and thrombophlebitis (1-12/94).

The usual initial adult dose is 30 mg/m^2 weekly. Vinorelbine tartrate has also been given with cisplatin. Dose reduction is not required for renal insufficiency but is needed for hematologic toxicity or hepatic insufficiency. Safety and efficacy in children have not been established (1-12/94).

Stability— Vinorelbine tartrate injection is a colorless to pale yellow clear solution. Intact vials should be refrigerated at 2 to 8 °C and protected from light (by storage in the carton) and freezing. Intact vials are stable at room temperature (up to 25 °C) for up to 72 hours (1-12/94).

When diluted to 1.5 to 3 mg/ml in polypropylene syringes or to 0.5 to 2 mg/ml in PVC infusion containers, vinorelbine tartrate is stable for 24 hours at 5 to 30 °C with exposure to normal room light (1-12/94).

Sorption— Vinorelbine tartrate (Pierre Fabre) 50 mg/250 ml in dextrose 5% in water or sodium chloride 0.9% in PVC bags was infused through PVC sets over two hours at 2.08 ml/min at 22 °C with protection from light. HPLC analysis of the effluent solution found no loss due to sorption to plastic (1631).

Compatibility Information

Solution Compatibility

Vinorelbine tartrate

Solution	*Mfr*	*Mfr*	*Conc/L*	*Remarks*	*Ref*	*C/I*
Dextrose 5% in water	[a]		500 mg	Little or no loss by HPLC in 7 days at 4 °C protected from light	1631	C
Sodium chloride 0.9%	[a]		500 mg	4% loss in 3 days and 14% loss in 7 days by HPLC at 4 °C protected from light	1631	C

[a]Tested in PVC containers.

Y-Site Injection Compatibility (1:1 Mixture)

Vinorelbine tartrate

Drug	*Mfr*	*Conc*	*Mfr*	*Conc*	*Remarks*	*Ref*	*C/I*
Acyclovir sodium	BW	7 mg/ml[a]	BW	1 mg/ml[a]	Heavy white precipitate forms immediately	1558	I
Allopurinol sodium	BW	3 mg/ml[a]	BW	1 mg/ml[a]	Heavy gelatinous white precipitate forms immediately	1686	I
Amikacin sulfate	BR	5 mg/ml[a]	BW	1 mg/ml[a]	Physically compatible with no change in measured turbidity or increase in particle content in 4 hr at 22 °C under fluorescent light	1558	C
Aminophylline	AB	2.5 mg/ml[a]	BW	1 mg/ml[a]	Initial light haze becomes visible in room light along with large particles in 1 hr	1558	I
Amphotericin B	SQ	0.6 mg/ml[b]	BW	1 mg/ml[a]	Heavy yellow precipitate forms immediately	1558	I
Ampicillin sodium	WY	20 mg/ml[a]	BW	1 mg/ml[a]	Tiny particles form immediately, becoming large white particles in cloudy solution in 1 hr	1558	I
Aztreonam	SQ	40 mg/ml[a]	BW	1 mg/ml[a]	Physically compatible with no change in measured turbidity or increase in particle content in 4 hr at 22 °C under fluorescent light	1558	C
Bleomycin sulfate	BR	1 unit/ml[a]	BW	1 mg/ml[a]	Physically compatible with no change in measured turbidity or increase in particle content in 4 hr at 22 °C under fluorescent light	1558	C
Bumetanide	RC	0.04 mg/ml[a]	BW	1 mg/ml[a]	Physically compatible with no change in measured turbidity or increase in particle content in 4 hr at 22 °C under fluorescent light	1558	C

Vinorelbine tartrate

Drug	*Mfr*	*Conc*	*Mfr*	*Conc*	*Remarks*	*Ref*	*C/I*
Buprenorphine HCl	RKC	0.04 mg/ml[a]	BW	1 mg/ml[a]	Physically compatible with no change in measured turbidity or increase in particle content in 4 hr at 22 °C under fluorescent light	1558	**C**
Butorphanol tartrate	BR	0.04 mg/ml[a]	BW	1 mg/ml[a]	Physically compatible with no change in measured turbidity or increase in particle content in 4 hr at 22 °C under fluorescent light	1558	**C**
Calcium gluconate	AMR	40 mg/ml[a]	BW	1 mg/ml[a]	Physically compatible with no change in measured turbidity or increase in particle content in 4 hr at 22 °C under fluorescent light	1558	**C**
Carboplatin	BR	5 mg/ml[a]	BW	1 mg/ml[a]	Physically compatible with no change in measured turbidity or increase in particle content in 4 hr at 22 °C under fluorescent light	1558	**C**
Carmustine	BR	1.5 mg/ml[a]	BW	1 mg/ml[a]	Physically compatible with no change in measured turbidity or increase in particle content in 4 hr at 22 °C under fluorescent light	1558	**C**
Cefazolin sodium	GEM	20 mg/ml[a]	BW	1 mg/ml[a]	Large increase in measured turbidity occurs immediately and grows over 4 hr at 22 °C under fluorescent light	1558	**I**
Cefoperazone sodium	RR	40 mg/ml[a]	BW	1 mg/ml[a]	Heavy white flocculent precipitate forms immediately	1558	**I**
Cefotaxime sodium	HO	20 mg/ml[a]	BW	1 mg/ml[a]	Physically compatible with no change in measured turbidity or increase in particle content in 4 hr at 22 °C under fluorescent light	1558	**C**
Cefotetan disodium	STU	20 mg/ml[a]	BW	1 mg/ml[a]	Tiny particles form immediately, becoming numerous in cloudy solution in 4 hr at 22 °C under fluorescent light	1558	**I**
Ceftazidime	LI	40 mg/ml[a]	BW	1 mg/ml[a]	Physically compatible with no change in measured turbidity or increase in particle content in 4 hr at 22 °C under fluorescent light	1558	**C**
Ceftizoxime sodium	FUJ	20 mg/ml[a]	BW	1 mg/ml[a]	Physically compatible with no change in measured turbidity or increase in particle content in 4 hr at 22 °C under fluorescent light	1558	**C**
Ceftriaxone sodium	RC	20 mg/ml[a]	BW	1 mg/ml[a]	Physically compatible with no change in measured turbidity or increase in particle content in 4 hr at 22 °C under fluorescent light	1558	**C**
Cefuroxime sodium	GL	20 mg/ml[a]	BW	1 mg/ml[a]	Large increase in measured turbidity occurs immediately and grows over 4 hr at 22 °C under fluorescent light	1558	**I**

Vinorelbine tartrate

Drug	*Mfr*	*Conc*	*Mfr*	*Conc*	*Remarks*	*Ref*	*C/I*
Chlorpromazine HCl	RU	2 mg/ml[a]	BW	1 mg/ml[a]	Physically compatible with no change in measured turbidity or increase in particle content in 4 hr at 22 °C under fluorescent light	1558	C
Cimetidine HCl	SKB	12 mg/ml[a]	BW	1 mg/ml[a]	Physically compatible with no change in measured turbidity or increase in particle content in 4 hr at 22 °C under fluorescent light	1558	C
Cisplatin	BR	1 mg/ml	BW	1 mg/ml[a]	Physically compatible with no change in measured turbidity or increase in particle content in 4 hr at 22 °C under fluorescent light	1558	C
Clindamycin phosphate	AB	10 mg/ml[a]	BW	1 mg/ml[a]	Physically compatible with no change in measured turbidity or increase in particle content in 4 hr at 22 °C under fluorescent light	1558	C
Cyclophosphamide	MJ	10 mg/ml[a]	BW	1 mg/ml[a]	Physically compatible with no change in measured turbidity or increase in particle content in 4 hr at 22 °C under fluorescent light	1558	C
Cytarabine	CET	50 mg/ml	BW	1 mg/ml[a]	Physically compatible with no change in measured turbidity or increase in particle content in 4 hr at 22 °C under fluorescent light	1558	C
Dacarbazine	MI	4 mg/ml[a]	BW	1 mg/ml[a]	Physically compatible with no change in measured turbidity or increase in particle content in 4 hr at 22 °C under fluorescent light	1558	C
Dactinomycin	MSD	0.01 mg/ml[a]	BW	1 mg/ml[a]	Physically compatible with no change in measured turbidity or increase in particle content in 4 hr at 22 °C under fluorescent light	1558	C
Daunorubicin HCl	WY	1 mg/ml[a]	BW	1 mg/ml[a]	Physically compatible with little change in measured turbidity or increase in particle content in 4 hr at 22 °C under fluorescent light	1558	C
Dexamethasone sodium phosphate	LY	1 mg/ml[a]	BW	1 mg/ml[a]	Physically compatible with no change in measured turbidity or increase in particle content in 4 hr at 22 °C under fluorescent light	1558	C
Diphenhydramine HCl	ES	2 mg/ml[a]	BW	1 mg/ml[a]	Physically compatible with no change in measured turbidity or increase in particle content in 4 hr at 22 °C under fluorescent light	1558	C
Doxorubicin HCl	CET	2 mg/ml	BW	1 mg/ml[a]	Physically compatible with no change in measured turbidity or increase in particle content in 4 hr at 22 °C under fluorescent light	1558	C

Vinorelbine tartrate

Drug	*Mfr*	*Conc*	*Mfr*	*Conc*	*Remarks*	*Ref*	*C/I*
Doxycycline hyclate	ES	1 mg/ml[a]	BW	1 mg/ml[a]	Physically compatible with no change in measured turbidity or increase in particle content in 4 hr at 22 °C under fluorescent light	1558	C
Droperidol	JN	0.4 mg/ml[a]	BW	1 mg/ml[a]	Physically compatible with no change in measured turbidity or increase in particle content in 4 hr at 22 °C under fluorescent light	1558	C
Enalaprilat	MSD	0.1 mg/ml[a]	BW	1 mg/ml[a]	Physically compatible with no change in measured turbidity or increase in particle content in 4 hr at 22 °C under fluorescent light	1558	C
Etoposide	BR	0.4 mg/ml[a]	BW	1 mg/ml[a]	Physically compatible with no change in measured turbidity or increase in particle content in 4 hr at 22 °C under fluorescent light	1558	C
Famotidine	MSD	2 mg/ml[a]	BW	1 mg/ml[a]	Physically compatible with no change in measured turbidity or increase in particle content in 4 hr at 22 °C under fluorescent light	1558	C
Filgrastim	AMG	30 μg/ml[c]	BW	1 mg/ml[a]	Physically compatible with no change in measured turbidity or increase in particle content in 4 hr at 22 °C under fluorescent light	1687	C
Floxuridine	RC	3 mg/ml[a]	BW	1 mg/ml[a]	Physically compatible with no change in measured turbidity or increase in particle content in 4 hr at 22 °C under fluorescent light	1558	C
Fluconazole	RR	2 mg/ml	BW	1 mg/ml[a]	Physically compatible with no change in measured turbidity or increase in particle content in 4 hr at 22 °C under fluorescent light	1558	C
Fludarabine phosphate	BX	1 mg/ml[a]	BW	1 mg/ml[a]	Physically compatible with no change in measured turbidity or increase in particle content in 4 hr at 22 °C under fluorescent light	1558	C
Fluorouracil	RC	16 mg/ml[a]	BW	1 mg/ml[a]	Heavy white precipitate forms immediately	1558	I
Furosemide	ES	3 mg/ml[a]	BW	1 mg/ml[a]	Heavy white precipitate forms immediately	1558	I
Gallium nitrate	FUJ	0.4 mg/ml[a]	BW	1 mg/ml[a]	Physically compatible with no change in measured turbidity or increase in particle content in 4 hr at 22 °C under fluorescent light	1558	C
Ganciclovir sodium	SY	20 mg/ml[a]	BW	1 mg/ml[a]	White turbid solution with precipitate forms immediately	1558	I
Gentamicin sulfate	ES	5 mg/ml[a]	BW	1 mg/ml[a]	Physically compatible with no change in measured turbidity or increase in particle content in 4 hr at 22 °C under fluorescent light	1558	C

Vinorelbine tartrate

Drug	*Mfr*	*Conc*	*Mfr*	*Conc*	*Remarks*	*Ref*	*C/I*
Haloperidol lactate	MN	0.2 mg/ml[a]	BW	1 mg/ml[a]	Physically compatible with no change in measured turbidity or increase in particle content in 4 hr at 22 °C under fluorescent light	1558	C
Heparin sodium	ES	100 units/ml[a]	BW	1 mg/ml[a]	Physically compatible with no change in measured turbidity or increase in particle content in 4 hr at 22 °C under fluorescent light	1558	C
Hydrocortisone sodium phosphate	MSD	1 mg/ml[a]	BW	1 mg/ml[a]	Physically compatible with no change in measured turbidity or increase in particle content in 4 hr at 22 °C under fluorescent light	1558	C
Hydrocortisone sodium succinate	UP	1 mg/ml[a]	BW	1 mg/ml[a]	Physically compatible with no change in measured turbidity or increase in particle content in 4 hr at 22 °C under fluorescent light	1558	C
Hydromorphone HCl	KN	0.5 mg/ml[a]	BW	1 mg/ml[a]	Physically compatible with no change in measured turbidity or increase in particle content in 4 hr at 22 °C under fluorescent light	1558	C
Hydroxyzine HCl	ES	4 mg/ml[a]	BW	1 mg/ml[a]	Physically compatible with no change in measured turbidity or increase in particle content in 4 hr at 22 °C under fluorescent light	1558	C
Idarubicin HCl	AD	0.5 mg/ml[a]	BW	1 mg/ml[a]	Increase in measured turbidity no greater than dilution of idarubicin with sodium chloride 0.9%. No increase in particle content in 4 hr at 22 °C under fluorescent light	1558; 1675	C
Ifosfamide	MJ	25 mg/ml[a]	BW	1 mg/ml[a]	Physically compatible with no change in measured turbidity or increase in particle content in 4 hr at 22 °C under fluorescent light	1558	C
Imipenem–cilastatin sodium	MSD	10 mg/ml[a]	BW	1 mg/ml[a]	Physically compatible with no change in measured turbidity or increase in particle content in 4 hr at 22 °C under fluorescent light	1558	C
Lorazepam	WY	0.1 mg/ml[a]	BW	1 mg/ml[a]	Physically compatible with no change in measured turbidity or increase in particle content in 4 hr at 22 °C under fluorescent light	1558	C
Mannitol	BA	15%	BW	1 mg/ml[a]	Physically compatible with no change in measured turbidity or increase in particle content in 4 hr at 22 °C under fluorescent light	1558	C
Mechlorethamine HCl	MSD	1 mg/ml	BW	1 mg/ml[a]	Physically compatible with no change in measured turbidity or increase in particle content in 4 hr at 22 °C under fluorescent light	1558	C

Vinorelbine tartrate

Drug	*Mfr*	*Conc*	*Mfr*	*Conc*	*Remarks*	*Ref*	***C/I***
Melphalan	BW	0.1 mg/ml[a]	BW	1 mg/ml[a]	Physically compatible with no change in measured turbidity or increase in particle content in 4 hr at 22 °C under fluorescent light	1558	**C**
Meperidine HCl	WY	4 mg/ml[a]	BW	1 mg/ml[a]	Physically compatible with no change in measured turbidity or increase in particle content in 4 hr at 22 °C under fluorescent light	1558	**C**
Mesna	MJ	10 mg/ml[a]	BW	1 mg/ml[a]	Physically compatible with no change in measured turbidity or increase in particle content in 4 hr at 22 °C under fluorescent light	1558	**C**
Methotrexate sodium	LE	15 mg/ml[a]	BW	1 mg/ml[a]	Physically compatible with no change in measured turbidity or increase in particle content in 4 hr at 22 °C under fluorescent light	1558	**C**
Methylprednisolone sodium succinate	AB	5 mg/ml[a]	BW	1 mg/ml[a]	Heavy white precipitate forms immediately	1558	**I**
Metoclopramide HCl	RB	5 mg/ml	BW	1 mg/ml[a]	Physically compatible with no change in measured turbidity or increase in particle content in 4 hr at 22 °C under fluorescent light	1558	**C**
Metronidazole	BA	5 mg/ml	BW	1 mg/ml[a]	Physically compatible with no change in measured turbidity or increase in particle content in 4 hr at 22 °C under fluorescent light	1558	**C**
Minocycline HCl	LE	0.2 mg/ml[a]	BW	1 mg/ml[a]	Physically compatible with no change in measured turbidity or increase in particle content in 4 hr at 22 °C under fluorescent light	1558	**C**
Mitomycin	BR	0.5 mg/ml	BW	1 mg/ml[a]	Color changes from pale blue to reddish purple in 1 hr	1558	**I**
Mitoxantrone HCl	LE	0.5 mg/ml[a]	BW	1 mg/ml[a]	Physically compatible with little change in measured turbidity or increase in particle content in 4 hr at 22 °C under fluorescent light	1558	**C**
Morphine sulfate	WI	1 mg/ml[a]	BW	1 mg/ml[a]	Physically compatible with no change in measured turbidity or increase in particle content in 4 hr at 22 °C under fluorescent light	1558	**C**
Nalbuphine HCl	AST	10 mg/ml	BW	1 mg/ml[a]	Physically compatible with no change in measured turbidity or increase in particle content in 4 hr at 22 °C under fluorescent light	1558	**C**
Netilmicin sulfate	SC	5 mg/ml[a]	BW	1 mg/ml[a]	Physically compatible with no change in measured turbidity or increase in particle content in 4 hr at 22 °C under fluorescent light	1558	**C**

Vinorelbine tartrate

Drug	*Mfr*	*Conc*	*Mfr*	*Conc*	*Remarks*	*Ref*	*C/I*
Ondansetron HCl	GL	1 mg/ml[a]	BW	1 mg/ml[a]	Physically compatible with no change in measured turbidity or increase in particle content in 4 hr at 22 °C under fluorescent light	1558	C
Piperacillin sodium	LE	40 mg/ml[a]	BW	1 mg/ml[a]	Heavy white turbidity forms immediately, becoming white flocculent precipitate in 4 hr at 22 °C under fluorescent light	1558	I
Plicamycin	MI	0.01 mg/ml[a]	BW	1 mg/ml[a]	Physically compatible with no change in measured turbidity or increase in particle content in 4 hr at 22 °C under fluorescent light	1558	C
Streptozocin	UP	40 mg/ml[a]	BW	1 mg/ml[a]	Physically compatible with no change in measured turbidity or increase in particle content in 4 hr at 22 °C under fluorescent light	1558	C
Teniposide	BR	0.1 mg/ml[c]	BW	1 mg/ml[c]	Physically compatible with no change in measured turbidity or increase in particle content in 4 hr at 23 °C under fluorescent light	1725	C
Thiotepa	LE	10 mg/ml[a]	BW	1 mg/ml[a]	Cloudy solution with particles forms immediately	1558	I
Ticarcillin disodium	BE	30 mg/ml[a]	BW	1 mg/ml[a]	Physically compatible with no change in measured turbidity or increase in particle content in 4 hr at 22 °C under fluorescent light	1558	C
Ticarcillin disodium–clavulanate potassium	SKB	31 mg/ml[a]	BW	1 mg/ml[a]	Physically compatible with no change in measured turbidity or increase in particle content in 4 hr at 22 °C under fluorescent light	1558	C
Tobramycin sulfate	LI	5 mg/ml[a]	BW	1 mg/ml[a]	Physically compatible with no change in measured turbidity or increase in particle content in 4 hr at 22 °C under fluorescent light	1558	C
Trimethoprim–sulfamethoxazole	ES	0.8 + 4 mg/ml[a]	BW	1 mg/ml[a]	Heavy white turbidity forms immediately, developing particles in 1 hr	1558	I
Vancomycin HCl	LY	10 mg/ml[a]	BW	1 mg/ml[a]	Physically compatible with no change in measured turbidity or increase in particle content in 4 hr at 22 °C under fluorescent light	1558	C
Vinblastine sulfate	LI	0.12 mg/ml[a]	BW	1 mg/ml[a]	Physically compatible with no change in measured turbidity or increase in particle content in 4 hr at 22 °C under fluorescent light	1558	C
Vincristine sulfate	LI	0.05 mg/ml[a]	BW	1 mg/ml[a]	Physically compatible with no change in measured turbidity or increase in particle content in 4 hr at 22 °C under fluorescent light	1558	C

Vinorelbine tartrate

Drug	*Mfr*	*Conc*	*Mfr*	*Conc*	*Remarks*	*Ref*	*C/I*
Zidovudine	BW	4 mg/ml[a]	BW	1 mg/ml[a]	Physically compatible with no change in measured turbidity or increase in particle content in 4 hr at 22 °C under fluorescent light	1558	**C**

[a]*Tested in sodium chloride 0.9%.*
[b]*Tested in both dextrose 5% in water and sodium chloride 0.9%.*
[c]*Tested in dextrose 5% in water.*

Additional Compatibility Information

Solutions— Vinorelbine tartrate, diluted to between 1.5 and 3 mg/ml in dextrose 5% in water or sodium chloride 0.9% for intravenous injection from a syringe, is reported to be stable for 24 hours at 5 to 30 °C when exposed to normal room light (1-12/94).

Vinorelbine tartrate injection, diluted to between 0.5 and 2 mg/ml for intravenous infusion, is reported to be stable for up to 24 hours at 5 to 30 °C when exposed to normal room light in the following infusion solutions (1-12/94):

Dextrose 5% in sodium chloride 0.45%
Dextrose 5% in water
Ringer's injection
Ringer's injection, lactated
Sodium chloride 0.45%
Sodium chloride 0.9%

Additions to Commercial Drug Monograph Tables

ACYCLOVIR SODIUM
AHFS 8:18
Handbook on Injectable Drugs pp. 4–8

Y-Site Injection Compatibility (1:1 Mixture)

Drug	Mfr	Conc	Acyclovir sodium Mfr	Acyclovir sodium Conc	Remarks	Ref	C/I
Teniposide	BR	0.1 mg/ml[a]	BW	7 mg/ml[a]	Physically compatible with no change in measured turbidity or increase in particle content in 4 hr at 23 °C under fluorescent light	1725	C

[a]*Tested in dextrose 5% in water.*

AMIKACIN SULFATE
AHFS 8:12.02
Handbook on Injectable Drugs pp. 13–24

Solution Compatibility

Solution	Mfr	Amikacin sulfate Mfr	Amikacin sulfate Conc/L	Remarks	Ref	C/I
Dextrose 10% in water	SO	BR	250 mg/ 21 ml[a]	Visually compatible with no amikacin loss by TDx in 30 days at 5 °C in the dark	1731	C
	SO	BR	500 mg/ 22 ml[a]	Visually compatible with no amikacin loss by TDx in 30 days at 5 °C in the dark	1731	C

[a]*Tested in glass vials as a concentrate.*

Y-Site Injection Compatibility (1:1 Mixture)

Drug	Mfr	Conc	Amikacin sulfate Mfr	Amikacin sulfate Conc	Remarks	Ref	C/I
Teniposide	BR	0.1 mg/ml[a]	BR	5 mg/ml[a]	Physically compatible with no change in measured turbidity or increase in particle content in 4 hr at 23 °C under fluorescent light	1725	C

[a]*Tested in dextrose 5% in water.*

AMINO ACID INJECTION
AHFS 40:20
Handbook on Injectable Drugs pp. 24–51

Additive Compatibility

Drug	Mfr	Conc/L	Amino acid injection Mfr	Amino acid injection Conc/L	Remarks	Ref	C/I
Ganciclovir sodium	SY	3 and 5 g		TPN #183 to #185[a]	Precipitate forms	1744	I
	SY	2 g		TPN #183[a]	Precipitate forms	1744	I

[a]*Refer to Appendix I for the composition of parenteral nutrition solutions.*

Y-Site Injection Compatibility (1:1 Mixture)

Drug	Mfr	Conc	Amino acid injection Mfr	Amino acid injection Conc[a]	Remarks	Ref	C/I
Ganciclovir sodium	SY	3 and 5 mg/ml		TPN #183 to #185[a]	Precipitate forms	1744	I
	SY	2 mg/ml		TPN #183[a]	Precipitate forms	1744	I
	SY	1 mg/ml[b]		TPN #183[a]	Visually compatible with no ganciclovir loss by HPLC in 3 hr at 24 °C under fluorescent light. Less than 10% amino acids loss by HPLC in 2 hr	1744	C
	SY	2 mg/ml[c]		TPN #184 and #185[a]	Visually compatible with no ganciclovir loss by HPLC in 3 hr at 24 °C under fluorescent light. Less than 10% amino acids loss by HPLC in 3 hr	1744	C

[a]Refer to Appendix I for the composition of parenteral nutrition solutions.
[b]Ganciclovir sodium concentration after mixing was 0.83 mg/ml.
[c]Ganciclovir sodium concentration after mixing was 1.4 mg/ml

AMINOPHYLLINE
AHFS 86:16
Handbook on Injectable Drugs pp. 52–62

Additive Compatibility

Drug	Mfr	Conc/L	Aminophylline Mfr	Aminophylline Conc/L	Test Soln	Remarks	Ref	C/I
Ceftriaxone sodium	RC	20 g	AMR	1 g	D5W, NS[a]	Yellow color forms immediately. 3 to 6% ceftriaxone loss and 8 to 12% aminophylline loss by HPLC in 24 hr	1727	I
	RC	20 g	AMR	4 g	D5W, NS[a]	Yellow color forms immediately. 15 to 20% ceftriaxone loss and 7 to 9% aminophylline loss by HPLC in 24 hr	1727	I
	RC	40 g	AMR	1 g	D5W, NS[a]	Yellow color forms immediately. 15 to 18% ceftriaxone loss and 1 to 3% aminophylline loss by HPLC in 24 hr	1727	I
Flumazenil	RC	20 mg	AMR	2 g	D5W[b]	Visually compatible with no flumazenil loss by HPLC in 24 hr at 23 °C under fluorescent light. Aminophylline not tested	1710	C

[a]Tested in polyolefin containers.
[b]Tested in PVC containers.

Y-Site Injection Compatibility (1:1 Mixture)

Drug	*Mfr*	*Conc*	*Mfr*	*Conc*	*Remarks*	*Ref*	*C/I*
			Aminophylline				
Teniposide	BR	0.1 mg/ml[a]	AB	2.5 mg/ml[a]	Physically compatible with no change in measured turbidity or increase in particle content in 4 hr at 23 °C under fluorescent light	1725	**C**

[a]Tested in dextrose 5% in water.

AMPHOTERICIN B
AHFS 8:12.04 and 84:04.08
Handbook on Injectable Drugs pp. 67–72

Solution Compatibility

Solution	*Mfr*	*Mfr*	*Conc/L*	*Remarks*	*Ref*	*C/I*
		Amphotericin B				
Dextrose 5% in water	BA[a]	SQ	0.2, 0.5, 1 g	Visually compatible and little or no amphotericin B loss by HPLC in 5 days at 4 and 25 °C. Normal turbidity observed at 1-g/L concentration	1728	**C**

[a]Tested in PVC containers.

Y-Site Injection Compatibility (1:1 Mixture)

Drug	*Mfr*	*Conc*	*Mfr*	*Conc*	*Remarks*	*Ref*	*C/I*
			Amphotericin B				
Teniposide	BR	0.1 mg/ml[a]	SQ	0.6 mg/ml[a]	Physically compatible with no change in measured turbidity or increase in particle content in 4 hr at 23 °C under fluorescent light	1725	**C**

[a]Tested in dextrose 5% in water.

AMPICILLIN SODIUM
AHFS 8:12.16
Handbook on Injectable Drugs pp. 72–86

Additive Compatibility

Drug	*Mfr*	*Conc/L*	*Mfr*	*Conc/L*	*Test Soln*	*Remarks*	*Ref*	*C/I*
			Ampicillin sodium					
Cefotiam HCl	TAK	20 g	GRU	20 g	W	Visually compatible with 4% or less loss of each drug by HPLC in 2 hr	1738	**C**

Y-Site Injection Compatibility (1:1 Mixture)

Ampicillin sodium

Drug	*Mfr*	*Conc*	*Mfr*	*Conc*	*Remarks*	*Ref*	*C/I*
Ofloxacin	HO	2.2 mg/ml	HO	21.3 mg/ml	Visually compatible with no loss of either drug by HPLC in 2 hr at room temperature	1734	C
Teniposide	BR	0.1 mg/ml[a]	WY	20 mg/ml[b]	Physically compatible with no change in measured turbidity or increase in particle content in 4 hr at 23 °C under fluorescent light	1725	C

[a]*Tested in dextrose 5% in water.*
[b]*Tested in sodium chloride 0.9%.*

AMPICILLIN SODIUM–SULBACTAM SODIUM
AHFS 8:12.16
Handbook on Injectable Drugs pp. 86–88

Solution Compatibility

Ampicillin sodium–sulbactam sodium

Solution	*Mfr*	*Mfr*	*Conc/L*	*Remarks*	*Ref*	*C/I*
Sodium chloride 0.9%	[a]	PF	20 + 10 g	Visually compatible with 10% ampicillin loss in 32 and 68 hr at 24 and 5 °C, respectively	1739	C

[a]*Tested in PVC containers.*

Additive Compatibility

Ampicillin sodium–sulbactam sodium

Drug	*Mfr*	*Conc/L*	*Mfr*	*Conc/L*	*Test Soln*	*Remarks*	*Ref*	*C/I*
Aztreonam	SQ	10 g	PF	20 + 10 g	NS[a]	Visually compatible with 10% ampicillin loss by HPLC in 30 hr at 24 °C and 94 hr at 5 °C. Other drugs stable for longer periods	1739	C

[a]*Tested in PVC containers.*

Y-Site Injection Compatibility (1:1 Mixture)

Ampicillin sodium–sulbactam sodium

Drug	*Mfr*	*Conc*	*Mfr*	*Conc*	*Remarks*	*Ref*	*C/I*
Teniposide	BR	0.1 mg/ml[a]	RR	20 + 10 mg/ml[b]	Physically compatible with no change in measured turbidity or increase in particle content in 4 hr at 23 °C under fluorescent light	1725	C

[a]*Tested in dextrose 5% in water.*
[b]*Tested in sodium chloride 0.9%.*

ATRACURIUM BESYLATE
AHFS 12:20
Handbook on Injectable Drugs pp. 97–100

Drugs in Syringe Compatibility

			Atracurium besylate				
Drug (in syringe)	*Mfr*	*Amt*	*Mfr*	*Amt*	*Remarks*	*Ref*	*C/I*
Sufentanil citrate		50 μg/ml	BW	10 mg/ml	Physically compatible and atracurium chemically stable for 24 hr at 5 and 25 °C	1694	**C**

ATROPINE SULFATE
AHFS 12:08.08
Handbook on Injectable Drugs pp. 100–105

Drugs in Syringe Compatibility

			Atropine sulfate				
Drug (in syringe)	*Mfr*	*Amt*	*Mfr*	*Amt*	*Remarks*	*Ref*	*C/I*
Sufentanil citrate	JN	50 μg/ml	LY	0.4 mg/ml	Physically compatible with no change in measured turbidity or increase in particle content in 24 hr at 23 °C under fluorescent light	1711	**C**

Y-Site Injection Compatibility (1:1 Mixture)

			Atropine sulfate				
Drug	*Mfr*	*Conc*	*Mfr*	*Conc*	*Remarks*	*Ref*	*C/I*
Sufentanil citrate	JN	12.5 μg/ml[a]	LY	0.4 mg/ml[a]	Physically compatible with no change in measured turbidity or increase in particle content in 24 hr at 23 °C under fluorescent light	1711	**C**

[a]*Tested in dextrose 5% in water.*

AZTREONAM
AHFS 8:12.07
Handbook on Injectable Drugs pp. 106–111

Solution Compatibility

		Aztreonam				
Solution	*Mfr*	*Mfr*	*Conc/L*	*Remarks*	*Ref*	*C/I*
Sodium chloride 0.9%	[a]	SQ	10 g	Visually compatible with no aztreonam loss by HPLC in 96 hr at 5 and 24 °C	1739	**C**

[a]*Tested in PVC containers.*

Additive Compatibility

			Aztreonam					
Drug	*Mfr*	*Conc/L*	*Mfr*	*Conc/L*	*Test Soln*	*Remarks*	*Ref*	*C/I*
Ampicillin sodium–sulbactam sodium	PF	20 + 10 g	SQ	10 g	NS[a]	Visually compatible with 10% ampicillin loss by HPLC in 30 hr at 24 °C and 94 hr at 5 °C. Other drugs stable for longer periods	1739	**C**

[a]*Tested in PVC containers.*

Y-Site Injection Compatibility (1:1 Mixture)

			Aztreonam				
Drug	*Mfr*	*Conc*	*Mfr*	*Conc*	*Remarks*	*Ref*	*C/I*
Ondansetron HCl	GL	0.03 and 0.3 mg/ml[a]	SQ	40 mg/ml[a]	Visually compatible with little or no loss of either drug by HPLC in 4 hr at 25 °C under fluorescent light	1732	**C**
Teniposide	BR	0.1 mg/ml[a]	SQ	40 mg/ml[a]	Physically compatible with no change in measured turbidity or increase in particle content in 4 hr at 23 °C under fluorescent light	1725	**C**

[a]*Tested in dextrose 5% in water.*

BLEOMYCIN SULFATE
AHFS 10:00
Handbook on Injectable Drugs pp. 115–121

Y-Site Injection Compatibility (1:1 Mixture)

			Bleomycin sulfate				
Drug	*Mfr*	*Conc*	*Mfr*	*Conc*	*Remarks*	*Ref*	*C/I*
Teniposide	BR	0.1 mg/ml[a]	BR	1 unit/ml[b]	Physically compatible with no change in measured turbidity or increase in particle content in 4 hr at 23 °C under fluorescent light	1725	**C**

[a]*Tested in dextrose 5% in water.*
[b]*Tested in sodium chloride 0.9%.*

BUMETANIDE
AHFS 40:28
Handbook on Injectable Drugs pp. 125–127

Y-Site Injection Compatibility (1:1 Mixture)

Drug	Mfr	Conc	Bumetanide Mfr	Bumetanide Conc	Remarks	Ref	C/I
Teniposide	BR	0.1 mg/ml[a]	RC	0.04 mg/ml[a]	Physically compatible with no change in measured turbidity or increase in particle content in 4 hr at 23 °C under fluorescent light	1725	C

[a]*Tested in dextrose 5% in water.*

BUPIVACAINE HCL
AHFS 72:00
Handbook on Injectable Drugs pp. 127–128

Solution Compatibility

Solution	Mfr	Bupivacaine HCl Mfr	Bupivacaine HCl Conc/L	Remarks	Ref	C/I
Sodium chloride 0.9%	AB	AST	1.25 g	Visually compatible with no bupivacaine loss by HPLC in 32 days at 3 °C in the dark and 23 °C exposed to light when stored in polypropylene syringes	1718	C

Drugs in Syringe Compatibility

Drug (in syringe)	Mfr	Amt	Bupivacaine HCl Mfr	Bupivacaine HCl Amt	Remarks	Ref	C/I
Sodium bicarbonate	AB	4%, 0.05 to 0.6 ml	AST, WI	0.25, 0.5[a], 0.75%[a]; 20 ml	Precipitate forms in 1 to 2 min up to 2 hr at lowest amount of bicarbonate	1724	I
		1.4%, 1.5 ml	BEL	0.5%[b], 20 ml	Little or no loss of epinephrine by HPLC in 7 days at room temperature. Bupivacaine not tested	1743	C
		4.2 and 8.4%, 1.5 ml	BEL	0.5%[b], 20 ml	5 to 7% epinephrine loss by HPLC in 7 days at room temperature. Bupivacaine not tested	1743	C

[a]*Tested with and without epinephrine HCl 1:200,000 added.*
[b]*Tested with epinephrine HCl 1:200,000 added.*

BUPRENORPHINE HCL
AHFS 28:08.12
Handbook on Injectable Drugs pp. 129–130

Y-Site Injection Compatibility (1:1 Mixture)

			Buprenorphine HCl				
Drug	*Mfr*	*Conc*	*Mfr*	*Conc*	*Remarks*	*Ref*	*C/I*
Teniposide	BR	0.1 mg/ml[a]	RKC	0.04 mg/ml[a]	Physically compatible with no change in measured turbidity or increase in particle content in 4 hr at 23 °C under fluorescent light	1725	C

[a]*Tested in dextrose 5% in water.*

BUTORPHANOL TARTRATE
AHFS 28:08.12
Handbook on Injectable Drugs pp. 130–133

Y-Site Injection Compatibility (1:1 Mixture)

			Butorphanol tartrate				
Drug	*Mfr*	*Conc*	*Mfr*	*Conc*	*Remarks*	*Ref*	*C/I*
Teniposide	BR	0.1 mg/ml[a]	BR	0.04 mg/ml[a]	Physically compatible with no change in measured turbidity or increase in particle content in 4 hr at 23 °C under fluorescent light	1725	C

[a]*Tested in dextrose 5% in water.*

CALCIUM GLUCONATE
AHFS 40:12
Handbook on Injectable Drugs pp. 140–149

Y-Site Injection Compatibility (1:1 Mixture)

			Calcium gluconate				
Drug	*Mfr*	*Conc*	*Mfr*	*Conc*	*Remarks*	*Ref*	*C/I*
Teniposide	BR	0.1 mg/ml[a]	AMR	40 mg/ml[a]	Physically compatible with no change in measured turbidity or increase in particle content in 4 hr at 23 °C under fluorescent light	1725	C

[a]*Tested in dextrose 5% in water.*

CARBOPLATIN
AHFS 10:00
Handbook on Injectable Drugs pp. 149–151

Y-Site Injection Compatibility (1:1 Mixture)

			Carboplatin				
Drug	*Mfr*	*Conc*	*Mfr*	*Conc*	*Remarks*	*Ref*	*C/I*
Teniposide	BR	0.1 mg/ml[a]	BR	5 mg/ml[a]	Physically compatible with no change in measured turbidity or increase in particle content in 4 hr at 23 °C under fluorescent light	1725	C

[a]*Tested in dextrose 5% in water.*

CARMUSTINE
(BCNU)
AHFS 10:00
Handbook on Injectable Drugs pp. 152–154

Y-Site Injection Compatibility (1:1 Mixture)

			Carmustine				
Drug	*Mfr*	*Conc*	*Mfr*	*Conc*	*Remarks*	*Ref*	*C/I*
Teniposide	BR	0.1 mg/ml[a]	BR	1.5 mg/ml[a]	Physically compatible with no change in measured turbidity or increase in particle content in 4 hr at 23 °C under fluorescent light	1725	C

[a]*Tested in dextrose 5% in water.*

CEFAZOLIN SODIUM
AHFS 8:12.06
Handbook on Injectable Drugs pp. 161–169

Y-Site Injection Compatibility (1:1 Mixture)

			Cefazolin sodium				
Drug	*Mfr*	*Conc*	*Mfr*	*Conc*	*Remarks*	*Ref*	*C/I*
Ondansetron HCl	GL	0.03 and 0.3 mg/ml[a]	LI	20 mg/ml[a]	Visually compatible with little or no loss of either drug by HPLC in 4 hr at 25 °C under fluorescent light	1732	C
Teniposide	BR	0.1 mg/ml[a]	MAR	20 mg/ml[a]	Physically compatible with no change in measured turbidity or increase in particle content in 4 hr at 23 °C under fluorescent light	1725	C

[a]*Tested in dextrose 5% in water.*

CEFONICID SODIUM
AHFS 8:12.06
Handbook on Injectable Drugs pp. 169–172

Y-Site Injection Compatibility (1:1 Mixture)

			Cefonicid sodium				
Drug	*Mfr*	*Conc*	*Mfr*	*Conc*	*Remarks*	*Ref*	*C/I*
Teniposide	BR	0.1 mg/ml[a]	SKB	20 mg/ml[a]	Physically compatible with no change in measured turbidity or increase in particle content in 4 hr at 23 °C under fluorescent light	1725	C

[a]*Tested in dextrose 5% in water.*

CEFOPERAZONE SODIUM
AHFS 8:12.06
Handbook on Injectable Drugs pp. 172–176

Y-Site Injection Compatibility (1:1 Mixture)

			Cefoperazone sodium				
Drug	*Mfr*	*Conc*	*Mfr*	*Conc*	*Remarks*	*Ref*	*C/I*
Teniposide	BR	0.1 mg/ml[a]	RR	40 mg/ml[a]	Physically compatible with no change in measured turbidity or increase in particle content in 4 hr at 23 °C under fluorescent light	1725	C

[a]*Tested in dextrose 5% in water.*

CEFOTAXIME SODIUM
AHFS 8:12.06
Handbook on Injectable Drugs pp. 176–180

Drugs in Syringe Compatibility

			Cefotaxime sodium				
Drug (in syringe)	*Mfr*	*Amt*	*Mfr*	*Amt*	*Remarks*	*Ref*	*C/I*
Ofloxacin	HO	200 mg	HO	2 g	Visually compatible with no loss of either drug by HPLC in 4 hr at room temperature	1735	C

Y-Site Injection Compatibility (1:1 Mixture)

			Cefotaxime sodium				
Drug	*Mfr*	*Conc*	*Mfr*	*Conc*	*Remarks*	*Ref*	*C/I*
Teniposide	BR	0.1 mg/ml[a]	HO	20 mg/ml[a]	Physically compatible with no change in measured turbidity or increase in particle content in 4 hr at 23 °C under fluorescent light	1725	C

Y-Site Injection Compatibility (1:1 Mixture) (Cont.)

Cefotaxime sodium

Drug	*Mfr*	*Conc*	*Mfr*	*Conc*	*Remarks*	*Ref*	*C/I*
Vancomycin HCl		12.5, 25, 30, 50 mg/ml[b]		100 mg/ml[b]	White precipitate forms immediately	1721	I
		5 mg/ml[b]		100 mg/ml[b]	No precipitate visually observed over 7 days at room temperature, but nonvisual incompatibility cannot be ruled out	1721	?

[a]*Tested in dextrose 5% in water.*
[b]*Tested in sterile water for injection.*

CEFOTETAN DISODIUM
AHFS 8:12.07
Handbook on Injectable Drugs pp. 181–183

Y-Site Injection Compatibility (1:1 Mixture)

Cefotetan disodium

Drug	*Mfr*	*Conc*	*Mfr*	*Conc*	*Remarks*	*Ref*	*C/I*
Teniposide	BR	0.1 mg/ml[a]	STU	20 mg/ml[a]	Physically compatible with no change in measured turbidity or increase in particle content in 4 hr at 23 °C under fluorescent light	1725	C

[a]*Tested in dextrose 5% in water.*

CEFOXITIN SODIUM
AHFS 8:12.07
Handbook on Injectable Drugs pp. 183–190

Y-Site Injection Compatibility (1:1 Mixture)

Cefoxitin sodium

Drug	*Mfr*	*Conc*	*Mfr*	*Conc*	*Remarks*	*Ref*	*C/I*
Teniposide	BR	0.1 mg/ml[a]	MSD	20 mg/ml[a]	Physically compatible with no change in measured turbidity or increase in particle content in 4 hr at 23 °C under fluorescent light	1725	C

[a]*Tested in dextrose 5% in water.*

CEFTAZIDIME
AHFS 8:12.06
Handbook on Injectable Drugs pp. 191–197

Y-Site Injection Compatibility (1:1 Mixture)

			Ceftazidime				
Drug	*Mfr*	*Conc*	*Mfr*	*Conc*	*Remarks*	*Ref*	*C/I*
Ondansetron HCl	GL	0.03 and 0.3 mg/ml[a]	LI	40 mg/ml[a]	Visually compatible with less than 10% loss of either drug by HPLC in 4 hr at 25 °C under fluorescent light	1732	C
Teniposide	BR	0.1 mg/ml[a]	LI	40 mg/ml[a]	Physically compatible with no change in measured turbidity or increase in particle content in 4 hr at 23 °C under fluorescent light	1725	C

[a]*Tested in dextrose 5% in water.*

CEFTIZOXIME SODIUM
AHFS 8:12.06
Handbook on Injectable Drugs pp. 197–200

Y-Site Injection Compatibility (1:1 Mixture)

			Ceftizoxime sodium				
Drug	*Mfr*	*Conc*	*Mfr*	*Conc*	*Remarks*	*Ref*	*C/I*
Teniposide	BR	0.1 mg/ml[a]	FUJ	20 mg/ml[a]	Physically compatible with no change in measured turbidity or increase in particle content in 4 hr at 23 °C under fluorescent light	1725	C

[a]*Tested in dextrose 5% in water.*

CEFTRIAXONE SODIUM
AHFS 8:12.06
Handbook on Injectable Drugs pp. 200–204

Solution Compatibility

		Ceftriaxone sodium				
Solution	*Mfr*	*Mfr*	*Conc/L*	*Remarks*	*Ref*	*C/I*
Dextrose 5% in water	MG	RC	10 and 40 g	Visually compatible with 5% or less ceftriaxone loss in 48 hr at 4 and 20 °C after 10 days storage at −15 °C in polypropylene syringes	1720	C
Sodium chloride 0.9%	BA	RC	10 and 40 g	Visually compatible with 5% or less ceftriaxone loss in 48 hr at 4 and 20 °C after 10 days storage at −15 °C in polypropylene syringes	1720	C

Additive Compatibility

Ceftriaxone sodium

Drug	*Mfr*	*Conc/L*	*Mfr*	*Conc/L*	*Test Soln*	*Remarks*	*Ref*	*C/I*
Aminophylline	AMR	1 g	RC	20 g	D5W, NS[a]	Yellow color forms immediately. 3 to 6% ceftriaxone loss and 8 to 12% aminophylline loss by HPLC in 24 hr	1727	I
	AMR	4 g	RC	20 g	D5W, NS[a]	Yellow color forms immediately. 15 to 20% ceftriaxone loss and 7 to 9% aminophylline loss by HPLC in 24 hr	1727	I
	AMR	1 g	RC	40 g	D5W, NS[a]	Yellow color forms immediately. 15 to 18% ceftriaxone loss and 1 to 3% aminophylline loss by HPLC in 24 hr	1727	I
Theophylline	BA[b]	4 g	RC	40 g		Yellow color forms immediately. 14% ceftriaxone loss and no theophylline loss by HPLC in 24 hr	1727	I

[a]*Tested in polyolefin containers.*
[b]*Tested in PVC containers.*

Y-Site Injection Compatibility (1:1 Mixture)

Ceftriaxone sodium

Drug	*Mfr*	*Conc*	*Mfr*	*Conc*	*Remarks*	*Ref*	*C/I*
Teniposide	BR	0.1 mg/ml[a]	RC	20 mg/ml[a]	Physically compatible with no change in measured turbidity or increase in particle content in 4 hr at 23 °C under fluorescent light	1725	C

[a]*Tested in dextrose 5% in water.*

CEFUROXIME SODIUM
AHFS 8:12.06
Handbook on Injectable Drugs pp. 204–208

Y-Site Injection Compatibility (1:1 Mixture)

Cefuroxime sodium

Drug	*Mfr*	*Conc*	*Mfr*	*Conc*	*Remarks*	*Ref*	*C/I*
Teniposide	BR	0.1 mg/ml[a]	GL	20 mg/ml[a]	Physically compatible with no change in measured turbidity or increase in particle content in 4 hr at 23 °C under fluorescent light	1725	C

[a]*Tested in dextrose 5% in water.*

CHLORPROMAZINE HCL
AHFS 28:16.08

Handbook on Injectable Drugs pp. 240–245

Y-Site Injection Compatibility (1:1 Mixture)

			Chlorpromazine HCl				
Drug	*Mfr*	*Conc*	*Mfr*	*Conc*	*Remarks*	*Ref*	*C/I*
Teniposide	BR	0.1 mg/ml[a]	SCN	2 mg/ml[a]	Physically compatible with no change in measured turbidity or increase in particle content in 4 hr at 23 °C under fluorescent light	1725	C

[a]*Tested in dextrose 5% in water.*

CIMETIDINE HCL
AHFS 56:40

Handbook on Injectable Drugs pp. 246–257

Solution Compatibility

		Cimetidine HCl				
Solution	*Mfr*	*Mfr*	*Conc/L*	*Remarks*	*Ref*	*C/I*
Sterile water for injection	AB	SKB	15 g	Visually compatible with 6% loss in 14 days and 10% loss in 28 days at 22 °C by HPLC. At 4 °C, 5% loss in 28 days and 14% loss in 56 days	1714	C

Additive Compatibility

			Cimetidine HCl					
Drug	*Mfr*	*Conc/L*	*Mfr*	*Conc/L*	*Test Soln*	*Remarks*	*Ref*	*C/I*
Flumazenil	RC	20 mg	SKB	2.4 g	D5W[a]	Visually compatible with no flumazenil loss by HPLC in 24 hr at 23 °C under fluorescent light. Cimetidine not tested	1710	C

[a]*Tested in PVC containers.*

Y-Site Injection Compatibility (1:1 Mixture)

			Cimetidine HCl				
Drug	*Mfr*	*Conc*	*Mfr*	*Conc*	*Remarks*	*Ref*	*C/I*
Teniposide	BR	0.1 mg/ml[a]	SKB	12 mg/ml[a]	Physically compatible with no change in measured turbidity or increase in particle content in 4 hr at 23 °C under fluorescent light	1725	C

[a]*Tested in dextrose 5% in water.*

CIPROFLOXACIN
AHFS 8:22
Handbook on Injectable Drugs pp. 257–261

Y-Site Injection Compatibility (1:1 Mixture)

		Ciprofloxacin					
Drug	*Mfr*	*Conc*	*Mfr*	*Conc*	*Remarks*	*Ref*	*C/I*
Teniposide	BR	0.1 mg/ml[a]	MI	2 mg/ml[a]	Physically compatible with no change in measured turbidity or increase in particle content in 4 hr at 23 °C under fluorescent light	1725	C

[a]*Tested in dextrose 5% in water.*

CISPLATIN
AHFS 10:00
Handbook on Injectable Drugs pp. 261–269

Y-Site Injection Compatibility (1:1 Mixture)

		Cisplatin					
Drug	*Mfr*	*Conc*	*Mfr*	*Conc*	*Remarks*	*Ref*	*C/I*
Teniposide	BR	0.1 mg/ml[a]	BR	1 mg/ml	Physically compatible with no change in measured turbidity or increase in particle content in 4 hr at 23 °C under fluorescent light	1725	C

[a]*Tested in dextrose 5% in water.*

CLINDAMYCIN PHOSPHATE
AHFS 8:12.28
Handbook on Injectable Drugs pp. 269–279

Solution Compatibility

		Clindamycin phosphate				
Solution	*Mfr*	*Mfr*	*Conc/L*	*Remarks*	*Ref*	*C/I*
Sterile water for injection	AB	AB	15 g	Visually compatible with no clindamycin loss by HPLC in 91 days at 4 and 22 °C	1714	C

Y-Site Injection Compatibility (1:1 Mixture)

		Clindamycin phosphate					
Drug	*Mfr*	*Conc*	*Mfr*	*Conc*	*Remarks*	*Ref*	*C/I*
Teniposide	BR	0.1 mg/ml[a]	AST	10 mg/ml[a]	Physically compatible with no change in measured turbidity or increase in particle content in 4 hr at 23 °C under fluorescent light	1725	C

[a]*Tested in dextrose 5% in water.*

CYCLOPHOSPHAMIDE
AHFS 10:00
Handbook on Injectable Drugs pp. 287–294

Y-Site Injection Compatibility (1:1 Mixture)

			Cyclophosphamide				
Drug	*Mfr*	*Conc*	*Mfr*	*Conc*	*Remarks*	*Ref*	*C/I*
Teniposide	BR	0.1 mg/ml[a]	MJ	10 mg/ml[a]	Physically compatible with no change in measured turbidity or increase in particle content in 4 hr at 23 °C under fluorescent light	1725	**C**

[a]*Tested in dextrose 5% in water.*

CYTARABINE
(CYTOSINE ARABINOSIDE)
AHFS 10:00
Handbook on Injectable Drugs pp. 296–301

Y-Site Injection Compatibility (1:1 Mixture)

			Cytarabine				
Drug	*Mfr*	*Conc*	*Mfr*	*Conc*	*Remarks*	*Ref*	*C/I*
Teniposide	BR	0.1 mg/ml[a]	CET	50 mg/ml	Physically compatible with no change in measured turbidity or increase in particle content in 4 hr at 23 °C under fluorescent light	1725	**C**

[a]*Tested in dextrose 5% in water.*

DACARBAZINE
AHFS 10:00
Handbook on Injectable Drugs pp. 301–303

Y-Site Injection Compatibility (1:1 Mixture)

			Dacarbazine				
Drug	*Mfr*	*Conc*	*Mfr*	*Conc*	*Remarks*	*Ref*	*C/I*
Teniposide	BR	0.1 mg/ml[a]	MI	4 mg/ml[a]	Physically compatible with no change in measured turbidity or increase in particle content in 4 hr at 23 °C under fluorescent light	1725	**C**

[a]*Tested in dextrose 5% in water.*

DACTINOMYCIN
(ACTINOMYCIN D)
AHFS 10:00

Handbook on Injectable Drugs pp. 303–305

Y-Site Injection Compatibility (1:1 Mixture)

			Dactinomycin				
Drug	*Mfr*	*Conc*	*Mfr*	*Conc*	*Remarks*	*Ref*	*C/I*
Teniposide	BR	0.1 mg/ml[a]	MSD	0.01 mg/ml[a]	Physically compatible with no change in measured turbidity or increase in particle content in 4 hr at 23 °C under fluorescent light	1725	**C**

[a]*Tested in dextrose 5% in water.*

DAUNORUBICIN HCL
AHFS 10:00

Handbook on Injectable Drugs pp. 305–308

Y-Site Injection Compatibility (1:1 Mixture)

			Daunorubicin HCl				
Drug	*Mfr*	*Conc*	*Mfr*	*Conc*	*Remarks*	*Ref*	*C/I*
Teniposide	BR	0.1 mg/ml[a]	WY	1 mg/ml[a]	Physically compatible with no change in measured turbidity or increase in particle content in 4 hr at 23 °C under fluorescent light	1725	**C**

[a]*Tested in dextrose 5% in water.*

DEXAMETHASONE SODIUM PHOSPHATE
AHFS 68:04

Handbook on Injectable Drugs pp. 308–313

Additive Compatibility

			Dexamethasone sodium phosphate					
Drug	*Mfr*	*Conc/L*	*Mfr*	*Conc/L*	*Test Soln*	*Remarks*	*Ref*	*C/I*
Diphenhydramine HCl with lorazepam and metoclopramide HCl	ES WY DU	2 g 40 mg 4 g	AMR	400 mg	NS[a]	Rapid lorazepam loss of 8, 10, and 15% at 3, 23, and 30 °C, respectively, in 24 hr by HPLC. Other drugs stable for 14 days by HPLC at all three storage temperatures	1733	**I**

[a]*Tested in Pharmacia-Deltec PVC pump reservoirs.*

Drugs in Syringe Compatibility

Dexamethasone sodium phosphate

Drug (in syringe)	*Mfr*	*Amt*	*Mfr*	*Amt*	*Remarks*	*Ref*	*C/I*
Sufentanil citrate	JN	50 µg/ml	AMR	4 mg/ml	Physically compatible with no change in measured turbidity or increase in particle content in 24 hr at 23 °C under fluorescent light	1711	**C**

Y-Site Injection Compatibility (1:1 Mixture)

Dexamethasone sodium phosphate

Drug	*Mfr*	*Conc*	*Mfr*	*Conc*	*Remarks*	*Ref*	*C/I*
Sufentanil citrate	JN	12.5 µg/ml[a]	AMR	1 mg/ml[a]	Physically compatible with no change in measured turbidity or increase in particle content in 24 hr at 23 °C under fluorescent light	1711	**C**
Teniposide	BR	0.1 mg/ml[a]	LY	1 mg/ml[a]	Physically compatible with no change in measured turbidity or increase in particle content in 4 hr at 23 °C under fluorescent light	1725	**C**

[a]*Tested in dextrose 5% in water.*

DIAZEPAM
AHFS 28:24.08
Handbook on Injectable Drugs pp. 321–328

Drugs in Syringe Compatibility

Diazepam

Drug (in syringe)	*Mfr*	*Amt*	*Mfr*	*Amt*	*Remarks*	*Ref*	*C/I*
Sufentanil citrate	JN	50 µg/ml	ES	5 mg/ml	White turbidity forms immediately. Precipitate forms in 24 hr at 23 °C	1711	**I**

Y-Site Injection Compatibility (1:1 Mixture)

Diazepam

Drug	*Mfr*	*Conc*	*Mfr*	*Conc*	*Remarks*	*Ref*	*C/I*
Sufentanil citrate	JN	12.5 µg/ml[a]	ES	0.5 mg/ml[a]	Physically compatible with no change in measured turbidity or increase in particle content in 24 hr at 23 °C under fluorescent light	1711	**C**

[a]*Tested in dextrose 5% in water.*

DIPHENHYDRAMINE HCL
AHFS 56:22
Handbook on Injectable Drugs pp. 338–342

Additive Compatibility

Diphenhydramine HCl

Drug	*Mfr*	*Conc/L*	*Mfr*	*Conc/L*	*Test Soln*	*Remarks*	*Ref*	*C/I*
Dexamethasone sodium phosphate with lorazepam and metoclopramide HCl	AMR WY DU	400 mg 40 mg 4 g	ES	2 g	NS[a]	Rapid lorazepam loss of 8, 10, and 15% at 3, 23, and 30 °C, respectively, in 24 hr by HPLC. Other drugs stable for 14 days by HPLC at all three storage temperatures	1733	I
Hydrocortisone sodium succinate	UP	500 mg	SCN	80 mg	D5W[b]	Physically compatible with no change in measured turbidity or increase in particle content in 24 hr at 23 °C under fluorescent light	1729	C
	UP	1 g	SCN	500 mg	D5W[b]	Physically compatible with no change in measured turbidity or increase in particle content in 24 hr at 23 °C under fluorescent light	1729	C

[a]*Tested in Pharmacia-Deltec PVC pump reservoirs.*
[b]*Tested in PVC containers.*

Drugs in Syringe Compatibility

Diphenhydramine HCl

Drug (in syringe)	*Mfr*	*Amt*	*Mfr*	*Amt*	*Remarks*	*Ref*	*C/I*
Sufentanil citrate	JN	50 μg/ml	SCN	50 mg/ml	Physically compatible with no change in measured turbidity or increase in particle content in 24 hr at 23 °C under fluorescent light	1711	C

Y-Site Injection Compatibility (1:1 Mixture)

Diphenhydramine HCl

Drug	*Mfr*	*Conc*	*Mfr*	*Conc*	*Remarks*	*Ref*	*C/I*
Hydrocortisone sodium succinate	UP	1 mg/ml[a]	SCN	0.16 mg/ml[a]	Physically compatible with no change in measured turbidity or increase in particle content in 24 hr at 23 °C under fluorescent light	1729	C
	UP	2 mg/ml[a]	SCN	1 mg/ml[a]	Physically compatible with no change in measured turbidity or increase in particle content in 24 hr at 23 °C under fluorescent light	1729	C
Sufentanil citrate	JN	12.5 μg/ml[a]	SCN	2 mg/ml[a]	Physically compatible with no change in measured turbidity or increase in particle content in 24 hr at 23 °C under fluorescent light	1711	C

Y-Site Injection Compatibility (1:1 Mixture) (Cont.)

Diphenhydramine HCl

Drug	*Mfr*	*Conc*	*Mfr*	*Conc*	*Remarks*	*Ref*	*C/I*
Teniposide	BR	0.1 mg/ml[a]	ES	2 mg/ml[a]	Physically compatible with no change in measured turbidity or increase in particle content in 4 hr at 23 °C under fluorescent light	1725	C

[a]*Tested in dextrose 5% in water.*

DOBUTAMINE HCL
AHFS 12:12
Handbook on Injectable Drugs pp. 349–357

Additive Compatibility

Dobutamine HCl

Drug	*Mfr*	*Conc/L*	*Mfr*	*Conc/L*	*Test Soln*	*Remarks*	*Ref*	*C/I*
Flumazenil	RC	20 mg	LI	2 g	D5W[a]	Visually compatible with no flumazenil loss by HPLC in 24 hr at 23 °C under fluorescent light. Dobutamine not tested	1710	C

[a]*Tested in PVC containers.*

DOPAMINE HCL
AHFS 12:12
Handbook on Injectable Drugs pp. 357–363

Additive Compatibility

Dopamine HCl

Drug	*Mfr*	*Conc/L*	*Mfr*	*Conc/L*	*Test Soln*	*Remarks*	*Ref*	*C/I*
Flumazenil	RC	20 mg	AB	3.2 g	D5W[a]	Visually compatible with 7% flumazenil loss by HPLC in 24 hr at 23 °C under fluorescent light. Dopamine not tested	1710	C

[a]*Tested in PVC containers.*

DOXORUBICIN HCL
AHFS 10:00
Handbook on Injectable Drugs pp. 366–373

Y-Site Injection Compatibility (1:1 Mixture)

			Doxorubicin HCl				
Drug	*Mfr*	*Conc*	*Mfr*	*Conc*	*Remarks*	*Ref*	*C/I*
Teniposide	BR	0.1 mg/ml[a]	CET	2 mg/ml	Physically compatible with no change in measured turbidity or increase in particle content in 4 hr at 23 °C under fluorescent light	1725	**C**

[a]*Tested in dextrose 5% in water.*

DOXYCYCLINE HYCLATE
AHFS 8:12.24
Handbook on Injectable Drugs pp. 373–375

Y-Site Injection Compatibility (1:1 Mixture)

			Doxycycline hyclate				
Drug	*Mfr*	*Conc*	*Mfr*	*Conc*	*Remarks*	*Ref*	*C/I*
Teniposide	BR	0.1 mg/ml[a]	LY	1 mg/ml[a]	Physically compatible with no change in measured turbidity or increase in particle content in 4 hr at 23 °C under fluorescent light	1725	**C**

[a]*Tested in dextrose 5% in water.*

DROPERIDOL
AHFS 28:16.08
Handbook on Injectable Drugs pp. 376–381

Y-Site Injection Compatibility (1:1 Mixture)

			Droperidol				
Drug	*Mfr*	*Conc*	*Mfr*	*Conc*	*Remarks*	*Ref*	*C/I*
Teniposide	BR	0.1 mg/ml[a]	JN	0.4 mg/ml[a]	Physically compatible with no change in measured turbidity or increase in particle content in 4 hr at 23 °C under fluorescent light	1725	**C**

[a]*Tested in dextrose 5% in water.*

ENALAPRILAT
AHFS 24:04
Handbook on Injectable Drugs pp. 384–388

Y-Site Injection Compatibility (1:1 Mixture)

			Enalaprilat				
Drug	*Mfr*	*Conc*	*Mfr*	*Conc*	*Remarks*	*Ref*	*C/I*
Teniposide	BR	0.1 mg/ml[a]	MSD	0.1 mg/ml[a]	Physically compatible with no change in measured turbidity or increase in particle content in 4 hr at 23 °C under fluorescent light	1725	C

[a]*Tested in dextrose 5% in water.*

EPINEPHRINE HCL
AHFS 12:12
Handbook on Injectable Drugs pp. 390–394

Drugs in Syringe Compatibility

			Epinephrine HCl				
Drug (in syringe)	*Mfr*	*Amt*	*Mfr*	*Amt*	*Remarks*	*Ref*	*C/I*
Sodium bicarbonate	AB	3 mEq/ 3 ml	ES	1:100,000[a], 30 ml	11% lidocaine loss in 1 week and 22% loss in 2 weeks at 25 °C by GC. 28% epinephrine loss by HPLC in 1 week at 25 °C	1712	I
	AB	3 mEq/ 3 ml	ES	1:100,000[a], 30 ml	6% lidocaine loss by GC in 4 weeks at 4 °C. 2% epinephrine loss in 1 week and 12% loss in 3 weeks at 4 °C by HPLC	1712	C
	LY	0.1 mEq/ml	AST	1:100,000[b]	25% epinephrine loss by HPLC in 1 week at room temperature. Lidocaine not tested	1713	I
	AST	8.4%, 2 ml	AST	1:200,000[c], 20 ml	Visually compatible for up to 5 hr at room temperature	1724	C
	AST	8.4%, 2 ml	AST	1:200,000[d], 20 ml	Haze clarifies with gentle agitation	1724	?
	AB	4%, 4 ml	AST	1:200,000[c], 20 ml	Visually compatible for up to 5 hr at room temperature	1724	C
	AB	4%, 4 ml	AST	1:200,000[d], 20 ml	Haze clarifies with gentle agitation	1724	?
	AB	4%, 0.05 to 0.6 ml	AST, WI	1:200,000[e], 20 ml	Precipitate forms in 1 to 2 min up to 2 hr at lowest amount of bicarbonate	1724	I
		1.4 and 8.4%, 1.5 ml	BEL	1:80,000[f], 20 ml	8% epinephrine loss by HPLC in 7 days at room temperature. Lidocaine not tested	1743	C
		4.2 and 8.4%, 1.5 ml	BEL	1:200,000[g], 20 ml	5 to 7% epinephrine loss by HPLC in 7 days at room temperature. Bupivacaine not tested	1743	C
		1.4%, 1.5 ml	BEL	1:200,000[g], 20 ml	Little or no loss of epinephrine by HPLC in 7 days at room temperature. Bupivacaine not tested	1743	C

[a]*Lidocaine HCl 2% with epinephrine HCl 1:100,000.*
[b]*Lidocaine HCl 1% with epinephrine HCl 1:100,000.*
[c]*Lidocaine HCl 1 and 1.5% with epinephrine HCl 1:200,000.*
[d]*Lidocaine HCl 2% with epinephrine HCl 1:200,000.*
[e]*Bupivacaine HCl 0.5 and 0.75% with epinephrine HCl 1:200,000.*
[f]*Lidocaine HCl 2% with epinephrine HCl 1:80,000.*
[g]*Bupivacaine HCl 0.5% with epinephrine HCl 1:200,000.*

ETOPOSIDE
AHFS 10:00
Handbook on Injectable Drugs pp. 410–414

Y-Site Injection Compatibility (1:1 Mixture)

			Etoposide				
Drug	*Mfr*	*Conc*	*Mfr*	*Conc*	*Remarks*	*Ref*	*C/I*
Teniposide	BR	0.1 mg/ml[a]	BR	0.4 mg/ml[a]	Physically compatible with no change in measured turbidity or increase in particle content in 4 hr at 23 °C under fluorescent light	1725	C

[a]*Tested in dextrose 5% in water.*

FAMOTIDINE
AHFS 56:40
Handbook on Injectable Drugs pp. 414–419

Additive Compatibility

			Famotidine					
Drug	*Mfr*	*Conc/L*	*Mfr*	*Conc/L*	*Test Soln*	*Remarks*	*Ref*	*C/I*
Flumazenil	RC	20 mg	MSD	80 mg	D5W[a]	Visually compatible with 3% flumazenil loss by HPLC in 24 hr at 23 °C under fluorescent light. Famotidine not tested	1710	C

[a]*Tested in PVC containers.*

Y-Site Injection Compatibility (1:1 Mixture)

			Famotidine				
Drug	*Mfr*	*Conc*	*Mfr*	*Conc*	*Remarks*	*Ref*	*C/I*
Teniposide	BR	0.1 mg/ml[a]	MSD	2 mg/ml[a]	Physically compatible with no change in measured turbidity or increase in particle content in 4 hr at 23 °C under fluorescent light	1725	C

[a]*Tested in dextrose 5% in water.*

FLOXURIDINE
AHFS 10:00
Handbook on Injectable Drugs pp. 444–446

Y-Site Injection Compatibility (1:1 Mixture)

Drug	Mfr	Conc	Floxuridine Mfr	Floxuridine Conc	Remarks	Ref	C/I
Teniposide	BR	0.1 mg/ml[a]	RC	3 mg/ml[a]	Physically compatible with no change in measured turbidity or increase in particle content in 4 hr at 23 °C under fluorescent light	1725	C

[a]*Tested in dextrose 5% in water.*

FLUCONAZOLE
AHFS 8:12.04
Handbook on Injectable Drugs pp. 446–451

Additive Compatibility

Drug	Mfr	Conc/L	Fluconazole Mfr	Fluconazole Conc/L	Test Soln	Remarks	Ref	C/I
Ranitidine HCl with ondansetron HCl	GL GL	500 mg 100 mg	RR	2 g	[a]	Visually compatible with no loss of any drug by HPLC in 4 hr	1730	C

[a]*Tested in PVC containers.*

Y-Site Injection Compatibility (1:1 Mixture)

Drug	Mfr	Conc	Fluconazole Mfr	Fluconazole Conc	Remarks	Ref	C/I
Ondansetron HCl	GL	0.03 and 0.3 mg/ml[a]	RR	2 mg/ml[b]	Visually compatible with little or no loss of either drug by HPLC in 4 hr at 25 °C under fluorescent light	1732	C
Ranitidine HCl	GL	0.5 and 2 mg/ml[a]	RR	2 mg/ml[b]	Visually compatible with no loss of either drug by HPLC in 4 hr	1730	C
Teniposide	BR	0.1 mg/ml[a]	RR	2 mg/ml	Physically compatible with no change in measured turbidity or increase in particle content in 4 hr at 23 °C under fluorescent light	1725	C

[a]*Tested in dextrose 5% in water.*
[b]*Tested in sodium chloride 0.9%.*

FLUDARABINE PHOSPHATE
AHFS 10:00
Handbook on Injectable Drugs pp. 452–456

Y-Site Injection Compatibility (1:1 Mixture)

			Fludarabine phosphate				
Drug	*Mfr*	*Conc*	*Mfr*	*Conc*	*Remarks*	*Ref*	*C/I*
Teniposide	BR	0.1 mg/ml[a]	BX	1 mg/ml[a]	Physically compatible with no change in measured turbidity or increase in particle content in 4 hr at 23 °C under fluorescent light	1725	C

[a]*Tested in dextrose 5% in water.*

FLUOROURACIL
(5-FLUOROURACIL)
AHFS 10:00
Handbook on Injectable Drugs pp. 457–464

Y-Site Injection Compatibility (1:1 Mixture)

			Fluorouracil				
Drug	*Mfr*	*Conc*	*Mfr*	*Conc*	*Remarks*	*Ref*	*C/I*
Teniposide	BR	0.1 mg/ml[a]	AD	16 mg/ml[a]	Physically compatible with no change in measured turbidity or increase in particle content in 4 hr at 23 °C under fluorescent light	1725	C

[a]*Tested in dextrose 5% in water.*

FOSCARNET SODIUM
AHFS 8:18
Handbook on Injectable Drugs pp. 466–470

Solution Compatibility

		Foscarnet sodium				
Solution	*Mfr*	*Mfr*	*Conc/L*	*Remarks*	*Ref*	*C/I*
Sodium chloride 0.9%	MG[a]	AST	12 g	Visually compatible and chemically stable by HPLC for 30 days at 25 °C in light or dark and at 5 °C in the dark	1726	C

[a]*Tested in PVC containers.*

FUROSEMIDE
(FRUSEMIDE)
AHFS 40:28
Handbook on Injectable Drugs pp. 470–479

Y-Site Injection Compatibility (1:1 Mixture)

			Furosemide				
Drug	*Mfr*	*Conc*	*Mfr*	*Conc*	*Remarks*	*Ref*	*C/I*
Labetalol HCl	SC	1.6 mg/ml[a]	ES	10 mg/ml[a]	White precipitate forms immediately	1714	I
Teniposide	BR	0.1 mg/ml[b]	AB	3 mg/ml[b]	Physically compatible with no change in measured turbidity or increase in particle content in 4 hr at 23 °C under fluorescent light	1725	C

[a]*Furosemide 0.5 ml injected in the Y-site port of a running infusion of labetalol HCl in dextrose 5% in water.*
[b]*Tested in dextrose 5% in water.*

GALLIUM NITRATE
AHFS 92:00
Handbook on Injectable Drugs pp. 479–481

Y-Site Injection Compatibility (1:1 Mixture)

			Gallium nitrate				
Drug	*Mfr*	*Conc*	*Mfr*	*Conc*	*Remarks*	*Ref*	*C/I*
Teniposide	BR	0.1 mg/ml[a]	FUJ	0.4 mg/ml[a]	Physically compatible with no change in measured turbidity or increase in particle content in 4 hr at 23 °C under fluorescent light	1725	C

[a]*Tested in dextrose 5% in water.*

GANCICLOVIR SODIUM
AHFS 8:18
Handbook on Injectable Drugs pp. 482–484

Solution Compatibility

		Ganciclovir sodium				
Solution	*Mfr*	*Mfr*	*Conc/L*	*Remarks*	*Ref*	*C/I*
Sodium chloride 0.9%	AB[a]	SY	5.8 g	3% or less ganciclovir loss in 10 days at 4 °C and no loss in 12 hr at 25 °C by HPLC	1742	C
TPN #183[b] (2-in-1)		SY	2 g	Precipitate forms	1744	I
TPN #183 to #185[b] (2-in-1)		SY	3 and 5 g	Precipitate forms	1744	I

[a]*Tested in polypropylene infusion pump syringes (Healthtek).*
[b]*Refer to Appendix I for the composition of parenteral nutrition solutions.*

Y-Site Injection Compatibility (1:1 Mixture)

Drug	Mfr	Conc	Ganciclovir sodium Mfr	Conc	Remarks	Ref	C/I
Teniposide	BR	0.1 mg/ml[a]	SY	20 mg/ml[a]	Physically compatible with no change in measured turbidity or increase in particle content in 4 hr at 23 °C under fluorescent light	1725	C
TPN #183[b] (2-in-1)			SY	2 mg/ml	Precipitate forms	1744	I
			SY	1 mg/ml[c]	Visually compatible with no ganciclovir loss by HPLC in 3 hr at 24 °C under fluorescent light. Less than 10% amino acids loss by HPLC in 2 hr	1744	C
TPN #183 to #185[b] (2-in-1)			SY	3 and 5 mg/ml	Precipitate forms	1744	I
TPN #184 and #185[b] (2-in-1)			SY	2 mg/ml[d]	Visually compatible with no ganciclovir loss by HPLC in 3 hr at 24 °C under fluorescent light. Less than 10% amino acids loss by HPLC in 3 hr	1744	C

[a]*Tested in dextrose 5% in water.*
[b]*Refer to Appendix I for the composition of parenteral nutrition solutions.*
[c]*Ganciclovir sodium concentration after mixing was 0.83 mg/ml.*
[d]*Ganciclovir sodium concentration after mixing was 1.4 mg/ml.*

GENTAMICIN SULFATE
AHFS 8:12.02

Handbook on Injectable Drugs pp. 484–497

Solution Compatibility

Solution	Mfr	Gentamicin sulfate Mfr	Conc/L	Remarks	Ref	C/I
Dextrose 10% in water	SO	SC	60 mg/ 21.5 ml[a]	Visually compatible with no gentamicin loss by TDx in 30 days at 5 °C in the dark	1731	C
	SO	SC	120 mg/ 23 ml[a]	Visually compatible with no gentamicin loss by TDx in 30 days at 5 °C in the dark	1731	C

[a]*Tested in glass vials as a concentrate.*

Y-Site Injection Compatibility (1:1 Mixture)

Drug	Mfr	Conc	Gentamicin sulfate Mfr	Conc	Remarks	Ref	C/I
Teniposide	BR	0.1 mg/ml[a]	LY	5 mg/ml[a]	Physically compatible with no change in measured turbidity or increase in particle content in 4 hr at 23 °C under fluorescent light	1725	C

[a]*Tested in dextrose 5% in water.*

HALOPERIDOL LACTATE
AHFS 28:16.08
Handbook on Injectable Drugs pp. 505–507

Solution Compatibility

Haloperidol lactate

Solution	*Mfr*	*Mfr*	*Conc/L*	*Remarks*	*Ref*	*C/I*
Dextrose 5% in sodium chloride 0.2%	AB	MN	0.1 to 1 g	Visually compatible for 7 days at 21 °C	1740	**C**
	AB	MN	2 and 3 g	Precipitate forms in 30 to 60 min	1740	**I**
Dextrose 5% in water	AB	MN	0.1 to 3 g	Visually compatible for 7 days at 21 °C	1740	**C**
Ringer's injection, lactated	AB	MN	0.1 to 1 g	Visually compatible for 7 days at 21 °C	1740	**C**
	AB	MN	2 g	Precipitate forms within 15 min	1740	**I**
	AB	MN	3 g	Precipitate forms immediately	1740	**I**
Sodium chloride 0.45%	AB	MN	0.1 to 1 g	Visually compatible for 7 days at 21 °C	1740	**C**
	AB	MN	2 g	Precipitate forms within 15 min	1740	**I**
	AB	MN	3 g	Precipitate forms immediately	1740	**I**
Sodium chloride 0.9%	AB	MN	0.1 to 0.75 g	Visually compatible for 7 days at 21 °C	1740	**C**
	AB	MN	1 to 3 g	Precipitate forms immediately	1740	**I**

Drugs in Syringe Compatibility

Haloperidol lactate

Drug (in syringe)	*Mfr*	*Amt*	*Mfr*	*Amt*	*Remarks*	*Ref*	*C/I*
Sufentanil citrate	JN	50 μg/ml	MN	5 mg/ml	Physically compatible with no change in measured turbidity or increase in particle content in 24 hr at 23 °C under fluorescent light	1711	**C**

Y-Site Injection Compatibility (1:1 Mixture)

Haloperidol lactate

Drug	*Mfr*	*Conc*	*Mfr*	*Conc*	*Remarks*	*Ref*	*C/I*
Sufentanil citrate	JN	12.5 μg/ml[a]	MN	0.2 mg/ml[a]	Physically compatible with no change in measured turbidity or increase in particle content in 24 hr at 23 °C under fluorescent light	1711	**C**
Teniposide	BR	0.1 mg/ml[a]	MN	0.2 mg/ml[a]	Physically compatible with no change in measured turbidity or increase in particle content in 4 hr at 23 °C under fluorescent light	1725	**C**

[a]*Tested in dextrose 5% in water.*

HEPARIN SODIUM
AHFS 20:12.04
Handbook on Injectable Drugs pp. 507–534

Additive Compatibility

			Heparin sodium					
Drug	*Mfr*	*Conc/L*	*Mfr*	*Conc/L*	*Test Soln*	*Remarks*	*Ref*	*C/I*
Flumazenil	RC	20 mg	ES	50,000 units	D5W[a]	Visually compatible with 4% flumazenil loss by HPLC in 24 hr at 23 °C under fluorescent light. Heparin not tested	1710	**C**

[a]*Tested in PVC containers.*

Y-Site Injection Compatibility (1:1 Mixture)

			Heparin sodium				
Drug	*Mfr*	*Conc*	*Mfr*	*Conc*	*Remarks*	*Ref*	*C/I*
Teniposide	BR	0.1 mg/ml[a]	ES	100 units/ ml[a]	Physically compatible with no change in measured turbidity or increase in particle content in 4 hr at 23 °C under fluorescent light	1725	**C**

[a]*Tested in dextrose 5% in water.*

HYDROCORTISONE SODIUM PHOSPHATE
AHFS 68:04
Handbook on Injectable Drugs pp. 542–545

Y-Site Injection Compatibility (1:1 Mixture)

			Hydrocortisone sodium phosphate				
Drug	*Mfr*	*Conc*	*Mfr*	*Conc*	*Remarks*	*Ref*	*C/I*
Teniposide	BR	0.1 mg/ml[a]	MSD	1 mg/ml[a]	Physically compatible with no change in measured turbidity or increase in particle content in 4 hr at 23 °C under fluorescent light	1725	**C**

[a]*Tested in dextrose 5% in water.*

HYDROCORTISONE SODIUM SUCCINATE
AHFS 68:04
Handbook on Injectable Drugs pp. 545–558

Additive Compatibility

			Hydrocortisone sodium succinate					
Drug	*Mfr*	*Conc/L*	*Mfr*	*Conc/L*	*Test Soln*	*Remarks*	*Ref*	*C/I*
Diphenhydramine HCl	SCN	80 mg	UP	500 mg	D5W[a]	Physically compatible with no change in measured turbidity or increase in particle content in 24 hr at 23 °C under fluorescent light	1729	**C**
	SCN	500 mg	UP	1 g	D5W[a]	Physically compatible with no change in measured turbidity or increase in particle content in 24 hr at 23 °C under fluorescent light	1729	**C**

[a]*Tested in PVC containers.*

Y-Site Injection Compatibility (1:1 Mixture)

			Hydrocortisone sodium succinate				
Drug	*Mfr*	*Conc*	*Mfr*	*Conc*	*Remarks*	*Ref*	*C/I*
Diphenhydramine HCl	SCN	0.16 mg/ml[a]	UP	1 mg/ml[a]	Physically compatible with no change in measured turbidity or increase in particle content in 24 hr at 23 °C under fluorescent light	1729	**C**
	SCN	1 mg/ml[a]	UP	2 mg/ml[a]	Physically compatible with no change in measured turbidity or increase in particle content in 24 hr at 23 °C under fluorescent light	1729	**C**
Teniposide	BR	0.1 mg/ml[a]	UP	1 mg/ml[a]	Physically compatible with no change in measured turbidity or increase in particle content in 4 hr at 23 °C under fluorescent light	1725	**C**

[a]*Tested in dextrose 5% in water.*

HYDROMORPHONE HCL
AHFS 28:08.08
Handbook on Injectable Drugs pp. 558–565

Additive Compatibility

			Hydromorphone HCl					
Drug	*Mfr*	*Conc/L*	*Mfr*	*Conc/L*	*Test Soln*	*Remarks*	*Ref*	*C/I*
Ondansetron HCl	GL	0.1 and 1 g	ES	0.5 g	NS[a]	Physically compatible with no change in measured turbidity or increase in particle content. Little or no loss of either drug by HPLC in 31 days at 4 and 22 °C and in 7 days at 32 °C	1745	**C**

[a]*Tested in PVC containers.*

Y-Site Injection Compatibility (1:1 Mixture)

Hydromorphone HCl

Drug	*Mfr*	*Conc*	*Mfr*	*Conc*	*Remarks*	*Ref*	*C/I*
Teniposide	BR	0.1 mg/ml[a]	KN	0.5 mg/ml[a]	Physically compatible with no change in measured turbidity or increase in particle content in 4 hr at 23 °C under fluorescent light	1725	C

[a]*Tested in dextrose 5% in water.*

HYDROXYZINE HCL
AHFS 28:24.92
Handbook on Injectable Drugs pp. 565–570

Drugs in Syringe Compatibility

Hydroxyzine HCl

Drug (in syringe)	*Mfr*	*Amt*	*Mfr*	*Amt*	*Remarks*	*Ref*	*C/I*
Sufentanil citrate	JN	50 μg/ml	ES	50 mg/ml	Physically compatible with no change in measured turbidity or increase in particle content in 24 hr at 23 °C under fluorescent light	1711	C

Y-Site Injection Compatibility (1:1 Mixture)

Hydroxyzine HCl

Drug	*Mfr*	*Conc*	*Mfr*	*Conc*	*Remarks*	*Ref*	*C/I*
Sufentanil citrate	JN	12.5 μg/ml[a]	ES	4 mg/ml[a]	Physically compatible with little change in measured turbidity or increase in particle content in 24 hr at 23 °C under fluorescent light	1711	C
Teniposide	BR	0.1 mg/ml[a]	WI	4 mg/ml[a]	Physically compatible with no change in measured turbidity or increase in particle content in 4 hr at 23 °C under fluorescent light	1725	C

[a]*Tested in dextrose 5% in water.*

IDARUBICIN HCL
AHFS 10:00
Handbook on Injectable Drugs pp. 570–573

Y-Site Injection Compatibility (1:1 Mixture)

Idarubicin HCl

Drug	*Mfr*	*Conc*	*Mfr*	*Conc*	*Remarks*	*Ref*	*C/I*
Teniposide	BR	0.1 mg/ml[a]	AD	0.5 mg/ml[a]	Unacceptable increase in turbidity occurs immediately	1725	I

[a]*Tested in dextrose 5% in water.*

IFOSFAMIDE
AHFS 10:00
Handbook on Injectable Drugs pp. 573–576

Y-Site Injection Compatibility (1:1 Mixture)

			Ifosfamide				
Drug	*Mfr*	*Conc*	*Mfr*	*Conc*	*Remarks*	*Ref*	***C/I***
Teniposide	BR	0.1 mg/ml[a]	MJ	25 mg/ml[a]	Physically compatible with no change in measured turbidity or increase in particle content in 4 hr at 23 °C under fluorescent light	1725	**C**

[a]*Tested in dextrose 5% in water.*

IMIPENEM–CILASTATIN SODIUM
AHFS 8:12.07
Handbook on Injectable Drugs pp. 577–581

Y-Site Injection Compatibility (1:1 Mixture)

			Imipenem–cilastatin sodium				
Drug	*Mfr*	*Conc*	*Mfr*	*Conc*	*Remarks*	*Ref*	***C/I***
Teniposide	BR	0.1 mg/ml[a]	MSD	10 mg/ml[b]	Physically compatible with no change in measured turbidity or increase in particle content in 4 hr at 23 °C under fluorescent light	1725	**C**

[a]*Tested in dextrose 5% in water.*
[b]*Tested in sodium chloride 0.9%.*

KETOROLAC TROMETHAMINE
AHFS 28:08.04
Handbook on Injectable Drugs pp. 611–612

Drugs in Syringe Compatibility

			Ketorolac tromethamine				
Drug (in syringe)	*Mfr*	*Amt*	*Mfr*	*Amt*	*Remarks*	*Ref*	***C/I***
Sufentanil citrate	JN	50 μg/ml	WY	30 mg/ml	Physically compatible with no change in measured turbidity or increase in particle content in 24 hr at 23 °C under fluorescent light	1711	**C**

Y-Site Injection Compatibility (1:1 Mixture)

			Ketorolac tromethamine				
Drug	*Mfr*	*Conc*	*Mfr*	*Conc*	*Remarks*	*Ref*	*C/I*
Sufentanil citrate	JN	12.5 µg/ml[a]	SY	1 mg/ml[a]	Physically compatible with no change in measured turbidity or increase in particle content in 24 hr at 23 °C under fluorescent light	1711	C

[a]*Tested in dextrose 5% in water.*

LABETALOL HCL
AHFS 24:08
Handbook on Injectable Drugs pp. 612–615

Y-Site Injection Compatibility (1:1 Mixture)

			Labetalol HCl				
Drug	*Mfr*	*Conc*	*Mfr*	*Conc*	*Remarks*	*Ref*	*C/I*
Furosemide	ES	10 mg/ml[a]	SC	1.6 mg/ml[a]	White precipitate forms immediately	1714	I

[a]*Furosemide 0.5 ml injected in the Y-site port of a running infusion of labetalol HCl in dextrose 5% in water.*

LEUCOVORIN CALCIUM
AHFS 92:00
Handbook on Injectable Drugs pp. 615–619

Y-Site Injection Compatibility (1:1 Mixture)

			Leucovorin calcium				
Drug	*Mfr*	*Conc*	*Mfr*	*Conc*	*Remarks*	*Ref*	*C/I*
Teniposide	BR	0.1 mg/ml[a]	LE	2 mg/ml[a]	Physically compatible with no change in measured turbidity or increase in particle content in 4 hr at 23 °C under fluorescent light	1725	C

[a]*Tested in dextrose 5% in water.*

LIDOCAINE HCL
(LIGNOCAINE HCL)
AHFS 24:04
Handbook on Injectable Drugs pp. 620–627

Additive Compatibility

			Lidocaine HCl					
Drug	*Mfr*	*Conc/L*	*Mfr*	*Conc/L*	*Test Soln*	*Remarks*	*Ref*	*C/I*
Flumazenil	RC	20 mg	AB	4 g	D5W[a]	Visually compatible with 4% flumazenil loss by HPLC in 24 hr at 23 °C under fluorescent light. Lidocaine not tested	1710	C

[a]*Tested in PVC containers.*

Drugs in Syringe Compatibility

Drug (in syringe)	Mfr	Amt	Lidocaine HCl Mfr	Amt	Remarks	Ref	C/I
Sodium bicarbonate	AB	3 mEq/ 3 ml	ES	2%[a], 30 ml	11% lidocaine loss in 1 week and 22% loss in 2 weeks at 25 °C by GC. 28% epinephrine loss by HPLC in 1 week at 25 °C	1712	I
	AB	3 mEq/ 3 ml	ES	2%[a], 30 ml	6% lidocaine loss by GC in 4 weeks at 4 °C. 2% epinephrine loss in 1 week and 12% loss in 3 weeks at 4 °C by HPLC	1712	C
	LY	0.1 mEq/ml	AST	1%[a], 30 ml	25% epinephrine loss by HPLC in 1 week at room temperature. Lidocaine not tested	1713	I
		0.088 mEq/ml		0.9%	11% lidocaine loss by fluorescence polarization immunoassay in 7 days at room temperature	1723	C
	AST	8.4%, 2 ml	AST	1 and 1.5%[b], 20 ml	Visually compatible for up to 5 hr at room temperature	1724	C
	AST	8.4%, 2 ml	AST	2%[b], 20 ml	Haze clarifies with gentle agitation	1724	?
	AB	4%, 4 ml	AST	1 and 1.5%[b], 20 ml	Visually compatible for up to 5 hr at room temperature	1724	C
	AB	4%, 4 ml	AST	2%[b], 20 ml	Haze clarifies with gentle agitation	1724	?
		1.4 and 8.4%, 1.5 ml	BEL	2%[c], 20 ml	8% epinephrine loss by HPLC in 7 days at room temperature. Lidocaine not tested	1743	C

[a]Tested with epinephrine HCl 1:100,000 added.
[b]Tested with and without epinephrine HCl 1:200,000 added.
[c]Tested with epinephrine HCl 1:80,000 added.

LORAZEPAM
AHFS 28:24.08
Handbook on Injectable Drugs pp. 630–633

Additive Compatibility

Drug	Mfr	Conc/L	Lorazepam Mfr	Conc/L	Test Soln	Remarks	Ref	C/I
Dexamethasone sodium phosphate with	AMR	400 mg	WY	40 mg	NS[a]	Rapid lorazepam loss of 8, 10, and 15% at 3, 23, and 30 °C, respectively, in 24 hr by HPLC. Other drugs stable for 14 days by HPLC at all three storage temperatures	1733	I
diphenhydramine HCl	ES	2 g						
and metoclopramide HCl	DU	4 g						

[a]Tested in Pharmacia-Deltec PVC pump reservoirs.

Drugs in Syringe Compatibility

			Lorazepam				
Drug (in syringe)	*Mfr*	*Amt*	*Mfr*	*Amt*	*Remarks*	*Ref*	*C/I*
Sufentanil citrate	JN	50 μg/ml	WY	2 mg/ml	Turbidity increases within 0.5 hr and continues to increase over 24 hr at 23 °C	1711	**I**

Y-Site Injection Compatibility (1:1 Mixture)

			Lorazepam				
Drug	*Mfr*	*Conc*	*Mfr*	*Conc*	*Remarks*	*Ref*	*C/I*
Sufentanil citrate	JN	12.5 μg/ml[a]	WY	0.1 mg/ml[a]	Large increase in measured turbidity occurs immediately and persists for 24 hr at 23 °C under fluorescent light	1711	**I**
Teniposide	BR	0.1 mg/ml[a]	WY	0.1 mg/ml[a]	Physically compatible with no change in measured turbidity or increase in particle content in 4 hr at 23 °C under fluorescent light	1725	**C**

[a]*Tested in dextrose 5% in water.*

MAGNESIUM SULFATE
AHFS 28:12.92
Handbook on Injectable Drugs pp. 633–639

Y-Site Injection Compatibility (1:1 Mixture)

			Magnesium sulfate				
Drug	*Mfr*	*Conc*	*Mfr*	*Conc*	*Remarks*	*Ref*	*C/I*
Morphine sulfate	[a]	2 mg/ml[b]	AB	2, 4, 8 mg/ml[b]	Visually compatible for 8 hr at room temperature	1719	**C**

[a]*Extemporaneously prepared product.*
[b]*Tested in sodium chloride 0.9%.*

MANNITOL
AHFS 36:40 and 40:28
Handbook on Injectable Drugs pp. 639–642

Y-Site Injection Compatibility (1:1 Mixture)

			Mannitol				
Drug	*Mfr*	*Conc*	*Mfr*	*Conc*	*Remarks*	*Ref*	*C/I*
Teniposide	BR	0.1 mg/ml[a]	WY	15%	Physically compatible with no change in measured turbidity or increase in particle content in 4 hr at 23 °C under fluorescent light	1725	**C**

[a]*Tested in dextrose 5% in water.*

MECHLORETHAMINE HCL
(MUSTINE HCL)
AHFS 10:00
Handbook on Injectable Drugs pp. 642–644

Y-Site Injection Compatibility (1:1 Mixture)

			Mechlorethamine HCl				
Drug	*Mfr*	*Conc*	*Mfr*	*Conc*	*Remarks*	*Ref*	*C/I*
Teniposide	BR	0.1 mg/ml[a]	MSD	1 mg/ml	Physically compatible with no change in measured turbidity or increase in particle content in 4 hr at 23 °C under fluorescent light	1725	**C**

[a]*Tested in dextrose 5% in water.*

MELPHALAN HCL
AHFS 10:00
Handbook on Injectable Drugs pp. 644–652

Y-Site Injection Compatibility (1:1 Mixture)

			Melphalan HCl				
Drug	*Mfr*	*Conc*	*Mfr*	*Conc*	*Remarks*	*Ref*	*C/I*
Teniposide	BR	0.1 mg/ml[a]	BW	0.1 mg/ml[a]	Physically compatible with no change in measured turbidity or increase in particle content in 4 hr at 23 °C under fluorescent light	1725	**C**

[a]*Tested in dextrose 5% in water.*

MEPERIDINE HCL
(PETHIDINE HCL)
AHFS 28:08.08
Handbook on Injectable Drugs pp. 653–662

Y-Site Injection Compatibility (1:1 Mixture)

			Meperidine HCl				
Drug	*Mfr*	*Conc*	*Mfr*	*Conc*	*Remarks*	*Ref*	*C/I*
Teniposide	BR	0.1 mg/ml[a]	WY	4 mg/ml[a]	Physically compatible with no change in measured turbidity or increase in particle content in 4 hr at 23 °C under fluorescent light	1725	**C**

[a]*Tested in dextrose 5% in water.*

MESNA
AHFS 92:00
Handbook on Injectable Drugs pp. 664–666

Y-Site Injection Compatibility (1:1 Mixture)

			Mesna				
Drug	*Mfr*	*Conc*	*Mfr*	*Conc*	*Remarks*	*Ref*	*C/I*
Teniposide	BR	0.1 mg/ml[a]	MJ	10 mg/ml[a]	Physically compatible with no change in measured turbidity or increase in particle content in 4 hr at 23 °C under fluorescent light	1725	C

[a]*Tested in dextrose 5% in water.*

METHOTREXATE SODIUM
AHFS 10:00
Handbook on Injectable Drugs pp. 680–687

Y-Site Injection Compatibility (1:1 Mixture)

			Methotrexate sodium				
Drug	*Mfr*	*Conc*	*Mfr*	*Conc*	*Remarks*	*Ref*	*C/I*
Teniposide	BR	0.1 mg/ml[a]	LE	15 mg/ml[a]	Physically compatible with no change in measured turbidity or increase in particle content in 4 hr at 23 °C under fluorescent light	1725	C

[a]*Tested in dextrose 5% in water.*

METHOTRIMEPRAZINE
AHFS 28:24.92
Handbook on Injectable Drugs pp. 687–688

Drugs in Syringe Compatibility

			Methotrimeprazine				
Drug (in syringe)	*Mfr*	*Amt*	*Mfr*	*Amt*	*Remarks*	*Ref*	*C/I*
Sufentanil citrate	JN	50 μg/ml	LE	20 mg/ml	Physically compatible with no change in measured turbidity or increase in particle content in 24 hr at 23 °C under fluorescent light	1711	C

Y-Site Injection Compatibility (1:1 Mixture)

			Methotrimeprazine				
Drug	*Mfr*	*Conc*	*Mfr*	*Conc*	*Remarks*	*Ref*	*C/I*
Sufentanil citrate	JN	12.5 μg/ml[a]	LE	0.2 mg/ml[a]	Physically compatible with no change in measured turbidity or increase in particle content in 24 hr at 23 °C under fluorescent light	1711	C

[a]*Tested in dextrose 5% in water.*

METHYLPREDNISOLONE SODIUM SUCCINATE
AHFS 68:04
Handbook on Injectable Drugs pp. 692–699

Y-Site Injection Compatibility (1:1 Mixture)

			Methylprednisolone sodium succinate				
Drug	*Mfr*	*Conc*	*Mfr*	*Conc*	*Remarks*	*Ref*	*C/I*
Teniposide	BR	0.1 mg/ml[a]	AB	5 mg/ml[a]	Physically compatible with no change in measured turbidity or increase in particle content in 4 hr at 23 °C under fluorescent light	1725	C

[a]*Tested in dextrose 5% in water.*

METOCLOPRAMIDE HCL
AHFS 56:40
Handbook on Injectable Drugs pp. 699–709

Additive Compatibility

			Metoclopramide HCl					
Drug	*Mfr*	*Conc/L*	*Mfr*	*Conc/L*	*Test Soln*	*Remarks*	*Ref*	*C/I*
Dexamethasone sodium phosphate with lorazepam and diphenhydramine HCl	AMR WY ES	400 mg 40 mg 2 g	DU	4 g	NS[a]	Rapid lorazepam loss of 8, 10, and 15% at 3, 23, and 30 °C, respectively, in 24 hr by HPLC. Other drugs stable for 14 days by HPLC at all three storage temperatures	1733	I

[a]*Tested in Pharmacia-Deltec PVC pump reservoirs.*

Drugs in Syringe Compatibility

			Metoclopramide HCl				
Drug (in syringe)	*Mfr*	*Amt*	*Mfr*	*Amt*	*Remarks*	*Ref*	*C/I*
Sufentanil citrate	JN	50 µg/ml	RB	5 mg/ml	Physically compatible with no change in measured turbidity or increase in particle content in 24 hr at 23 °C under fluorescent light	1711	C

Y-Site Injection Compatibility (1:1 Mixture)

			Metoclopramide HCl				
Drug	*Mfr*	*Conc*	*Mfr*	*Conc*	*Remarks*	*Ref*	*C/I*
Sufentanil citrate	JN	12.5 µg/ml[a]	RB	5 mg/ml	Physically compatible with no change in measured turbidity or increase in particle content in 24 hr at 23 °C under fluorescent light	1711	C

Y-Site Injection Compatibility (1:1 Mixture) (Cont.)

Metoclopramide HCl

Drug	*Mfr*	*Conc*	*Mfr*	*Conc*	*Remarks*	*Ref*	*C/I*
Teniposide	BR	0.1 mg/ml[a]	ES	5 mg/ml	Physically compatible with no change in measured turbidity or increase in particle content in 4 hr at 23 °C under fluorescent light	1725	**C**

[a]*Tested in dextrose 5% in water.*

METRONIDAZOLE
METRONIDAZOLE HCL
AHFS 8:40

Handbook on Injectable Drugs pp. 710–716

Additive Compatibility

Metronidazole

Drug	*Mfr*	*Conc/L*	*Mfr*	*Conc/L*	*Test Soln*	*Remarks*	*Ref*	*C/I*
Cefotiam HCl	TAK	2 g		500 mg/ 100 ml	[a]	Visually compatible with little or no loss of either drug by HPLC in 4 hr at room temperature	1737	**C**

[a]*Tested in metronidazole infusion.*

Y-Site Injection Compatibility (1:1 Mixture)

Metronidazole

Drug	*Mfr*	*Conc*	*Mfr*	*Conc*	*Remarks*	*Ref*	*C/I*
Teniposide	BR	0.1 mg/ml[a]	BA	5 mg/ml	Physically compatible with no change in measured turbidity or increase in particle content in 4 hr at 23 °C under fluorescent light	1725	**C**

[a]*Tested in dextrose 5% in water.*

MEZLOCILLIN SODIUM
AHFS 8:12.16

Handbook on Injectable Drugs pp. 717–720

Y-Site Injection Compatibility (1:1 Mixture)

Mezlocillin sodium

Drug	*Mfr*	*Conc*	*Mfr*	*Conc*	*Remarks*	*Ref*	*C/I*
Teniposide	BR	0.1 mg/ml[a]	MI	40 mg/ml[a]	Physically compatible with no change in measured turbidity or increase in particle content in 4 hr at 23 °C under fluorescent light	1725	**C**

[a]*Tested in dextrose 5% in water.*

MICONAZOLE
AHFS 8:12.04
Handbook on Injectable Drugs pp. 720–722

Y-Site Injection Compatibility (1:1 Mixture)

			Miconazole				
Drug	*Mfr*	*Conc*	*Mfr*	*Conc*	*Remarks*	*Ref*	*C/I*
Teniposide	BR	0.1 mg/ml[a]	JN	3.5 mg/ml[a]	Physically compatible with no change in measured turbidity or increase in particle content in 4 hr at 23 °C under fluorescent light	1725	C

[a]*Tested in dextrose 5% in water.*

MIDAZOLAM HCL
AHFS 28:24.08
Handbook on Injectable Drugs pp. 722–725

Solution Compatibility

		Midazolam HCl				
Solution	*Mfr*	*Mfr*	*Conc/L*	*Remarks*	*Ref*	*C/I*
Dextrose 5% in water	MG[a]	RC	0.5 g	Visually compatible with no midazolam loss by HPLC in 30 days at 23 °C in the dark or at 4 °C	1717	C
Sodium chloride 0.9%	MG[a]	RC	0.5 g	Visually compatible with no midazolam loss by HPC in 30 days at 23 °C in the dark or at 4 °C	1717	C

[a]*Tested in polyolefin containers.*

Drugs in Syringe Compatibility

			Midazolam HCl				
Drug (in syringe)	*Mfr*	*Amt*	*Mfr*	*Amt*	*Remarks*	*Ref*	*C/I*
Sufentanil citrate	JN	50 μg/ml	RC	5 mg/ml	Physically compatible with no change in measured turbidity or increase in particle content in 24 hr at 23 °C under fluorescent light	1711	C

Y-Site Injection Compatibility (1:1 Mixture)

			Midazolam HCl				
Drug	*Mfr*	*Conc*	*Mfr*	*Conc*	*Remarks*	*Ref*	*C/I*
Sufentanil citrate	JN	12.5 μg/ml[a]	RC	0.2 mg/ml[a]	Physically compatible with no change in measured turbidity or increase in particle content in 24 hr at 23 °C under fluorescent light	1711	C

[a]*Tested in dextrose 5% in water.*

MINOCYCLINE HCL
AHFS 8:12.24
Handbook on Injectable Drugs pp. 727–729

Y-Site Injection Compatibility (1:1 Mixture)

Minocycline HCl

Drug	*Mfr*	*Conc*	*Mfr*	*Conc*	*Remarks*	*Ref*	*C/I*
Teniposide	BR	0.1 mg/ml[a]	LE	0.2 mg/ml[a]	Physically compatible with no change in measured turbidity or increase in particle content in 4 hr at 23 °C under fluorescent light	1725	**C**

[a]*Tested in dextrose 5% in water.*

MITOMYCIN
AHFS 10:00
Handbook on Injectable Drugs pp. 730–734

Y-Site Injection Compatibility (1:1 Mixture)

Mitomycin

Drug	*Mfr*	*Conc*	*Mfr*	*Conc*	*Remarks*	*Ref*	*C/I*
Teniposide	BR	0.1 mg/ml[a]	BR	0.5 mg/ml	Physically compatible with no change in measured turbidity or increase in particle content in 4 hr at 23 °C under fluorescent light	1725	**C**

[a]*Tested in dextrose 5% in water.*

MITOXANTRONE HCL
AHFS 10:00
Handbook on Injectable Drugs pp. 734–736

Y-Site Injection Compatibility (1:1 Mixture)

Mitoxantrone HCl

Drug	*Mfr*	*Conc*	*Mfr*	*Conc*	*Remarks*	*Ref*	*C/I*
Teniposide	BR	0.1 mg/ml[a]	LE	0.5 mg/ml[a]	Physically compatible with no change in measured turbidity or increase in particle content in 4 hr at 23 °C under fluorescent light	1725	**C**

[a]*Tested in dextrose 5% in water.*

MORPHINE SULFATE
AHFS 28:08.08
Handbook on Injectable Drugs pp. 736–747

Additive Compatibility

			Morphine sulfate					
Drug	*Mfr*	*Conc/L*	*Mfr*	*Conc/L*	*Test Soln*	*Remarks*	*Ref*	*C/I*
Ondansetron HCl	GL	0.1 and 1 g	AST	1 g	NS[a]	Physically compatible with no change in measured turbidity or increase in particle content. Little or no loss of either drug by HPLC in 31 days at 4 and 22 °C and in 7 days at 32 °C	1745	C

[a]Tested in PVC containers.

Y-Site Injection Compatibility (1:1 Mixture)

			Morphine sulfate				
Drug	*Mfr*	*Conc*	*Mfr*	*Conc*	*Remarks*	*Ref*	*C/I*
Magnesium sulfate	AB	2, 4, 8 mg/ml[a]	[b]	2 mg/ml[a]	Visually compatible for 8 hr at room temperature	1719	C
Teniposide	BR	0.1 mg/ml[c]	AST	1 mg/ml[c]	Physically compatible with no change in measured turbidity or increase in particle content in 4 hr at 23 °C under fluorescent light	1725	C

[a]Tested in sodium chloride 0.9%.
[b]Extemporaneously prepared product.
[c]Tested in dextrose 5% in water.

NALBUPHINE HCL
AHFS 28:08.12
Handbook on Injectable Drugs pp. 764–767

Y-Site Injection Compatibility (1:1 Mixture)

			Nalbuphine HCl				
Drug	*Mfr*	*Conc*	*Mfr*	*Conc*	*Remarks*	*Ref*	*C/I*
Teniposide	BR	0.1 mg/ml[a]	DU	10 mg/ml	Physically compatible with no change in measured turbidity or increase in particle content in 4 hr at 23 °C under fluorescent light	1725	C

[a]Tested in dextrose 5% in water.

NETILMICIN SULFATE
AHFS 8:12.02
Handbook on Injectable Drugs pp. 770–776

Y-Site Injection Compatibility (1:1 Mixture)

			Netilmicin sulfate				
Drug	*Mfr*	*Conc*	*Mfr*	*Conc*	*Remarks*	*Ref*	*C/I*
Teniposide	BR	0.1 mg/ml[a]	SC	5 mg/ml[a]	Physically compatible with no change in measured turbidity or increase in particle content in 4 hr at 23 °C under fluorescent light	1725	**C**

[a]*Tested in dextrose 5% in water.*

OFLOXACIN
AHFS 8:22
Handbook on Injectable Drugs pp. 792–794

Drugs in Syringe Compatibility

			Ofloxacin				
Drug (in syringe)	*Mfr*	*Amt*	*Mfr*	*Amt*	*Remarks*	*Ref*	*C/I*
Cefotaxime sodium	HO	2 g	HO	200 mg	Visually compatible with no loss of either drug by HPLC in 4 hr at room temperature	1735	**C**

Y-Site Injection Compatibility (1:1 Mixture)

			Ofloxacin				
Drug	*Mfr*	*Conc*	*Mfr*	*Conc*	*Remarks*	*Ref*	*C/I*
Ampicillin sodium	HO	21.3 mg/ml	HO	2.2 mg/ml	Visually compatible with no loss of either drug by HPLC in 2 hr at room temperature	1734	**C**

ONDANSETRON HCL
AHFS 56:22
Handbook on Injectable Drugs pp. 794–800

Solution Compatibility

		Ondansetron HCl				
Solution	*Mfr*	*Mfr*	*Conc/L*	*Remarks*	*Ref*	*C/I*
Dextrose 5% in water	MG[a]	GL	0.03 and 0.3 g	Visually compatible with no ondansetron loss by HPLC in 14 days at 4 °C under fluorescent light and no microbial growth	1722	**C**

Solution Compatibility (Cont.)

Ondansetron HCl

Solution	*Mfr*	*Mfr*	*Conc/L*	*Remarks*	*Ref*	*C/I*
Sodium chloride 0.9%	MG[a]	GL	0.03 and 0.3 g	Visually compatible with no ondansetron loss by HPLC in 14 days at 4 °C under fluorescent light and no microbial growth	1722	**C**

[a]*Tested in Kraton polymer elastomeric infusion device (Homepump, Block).*

Additive Compatibility

Ondansetron HCl

Drug	*Mfr*	*Conc/L*	*Mfr*	*Conc/L*	*Test Soln*	*Remarks*	*Ref*	*C/I*
Fluconazole with ranitidine HCl	RR GL	2 g 500 mg	GL	100 mg	[a]	Visually compatible with no loss of any drug by HPLC in 4 hr	1730	**C**
Hydromorphone HCl	ES	0.5 g	GL	0.1 and 1 g	NS[a]	Physically compatible with no change in measured turbidity or increase in particle content. Little or no loss of either drug by HPLC in 31 days at 4 and 22 °C and in 7 days at 32 °C	1745	**C**
Morphine sulfate	AST	1 g	GL	0.1 and 1 g	NS[a]	Physically compatible with no change in measured turbidity or increase in particle content. Little or no loss of either drug by HPLC in 31 days at 4 and 22 °C and in 7 days at 32 °C	1745	**C**

[a]*Tested in PVC containers.*

Y-Site Injection Compatibility (1:1 Mixture)

Ondansetron HCl

Drug	*Mfr*	*Conc*	*Mfr*	*Conc*	*Remarks*	*Ref*	*C/I*
Aztreonam	SQ	40 mg/ml[a]	GL	0.03 and 0.3 mg/ml[a]	Visually compatible with little or no loss of either drug by HPLC in 4 hr at 25 °C under fluorescent light	1732	**C**
Cefazolin sodium	LI	20 mg/ml[a]	GL	0.03 and 0.3 mg/ml[a]	Visually compatible with little or no loss of either drug by HPLC in 4 hr at 25 °C under fluorescent light	1732	**C**
Ceftazidime	LI	40 mg/ml[a]	GL	0.03 and 0.3 mg/ml[a]	Visually compatible with less than 10% loss of either drug by HPLC in 4 hr at 25 °C under fluorescent light	1732	**C**
Fluconazole	RR	2 mg/ml[b]	GL	0.03 and 0.3 mg/ml[a]	Visually compatible with little or no loss of either drug by HPLC in 4 hr at 25 °C under fluorescent light	1732	**C**

Drug	Mfr	Conc	Ondansetron HCl Mfr	Ondansetron HCl Conc	Remarks	Ref	C/I
Paclitaxel	BR	0.3 mg/ml[a]	GL	0.03 and 0.3 mg/ml[a]	Visually compatible with no loss of either drug in 4 hr at 23 °C under fluorescent light	1741	C
	BR	1.2 mg/ml[a]	GL	0.03 and 0.3 mg/ml[a]	Visually compatible with no loss of either drug in 4 hr at 23 °C under fluorescent light	1741	C
Paclitaxel with ranitidine HCl	BR GL	1.2 mg/ml[a] 2 mg/ml[a]	GL	0.3 mg/ml[a]	Visually compatible with no loss of any drug by HPLC in 4 hr at 23 °C under fluorescent light	1741	C
Ranitidine HCl	GL	0.5 mg/ml[a]	GL	0.03, 0.1, 0.3 mg/ml[a]	Visually compatible with no loss of either drug by HPLC in 4 hr	1730	C
	GL	2 mg/ml[a]	GL	0.03, 0.1, 0.3 mg/ml[a]	Visually compatible with no loss of either drug by HPLC in 4 hr	1730	C
Teniposide	BR	0.1 mg/ml[a]	GL	1 mg/ml[a]	Physically compatible with no change in measured turbidity or increase in particle content in 4 hr at 23 °C under fluorescent light	1725	C

[a]Tested in dextrose 5% in water.
[b]Tested in sodium chloride 0.9%.

PACLITAXEL
AHFS 10:00
Handbook on Injectable Drugs pp. 808 813

Solution Compatibility

Solution	Mfr	Paclitaxel Mfr	Paclitaxel Conc/L	Remarks	Ref	C/I
Dextrose 5% in water	[a]	BR	0.2 to 0.58 g	Fluffy, white precipitate forms occasionally in administration set[b] just distal to pump chamber	1716	I
	MG[c]	BR	0.1 and 1 g	Physically compatible with no change in measured turbidity or increase in particle content in 3 days at 4, 22, and 32 °C. Small, needle-like crystals form after 3 days. Paclitaxel chemically stable by HPLC at 4, 22, and 32 °C until precipitation occurs	1746	C
Sodium chloride 0.9%	MG[c]	BR	0.1 and 1 g	Physically compatible with no change in measured turbidity or increase in particle content in 3 days at 4, 22, and 32 °C. Small, needle-like crystals form after 3 days. Paclitaxel chemically stable by HPLC at 4, 22, and 32 °C until precipitation occurs	1746	C

[a]Tested in glass bottles.
[b]Baxter polyethylene-lined administration set (Model 2C7552s) for the Flo-Gard 6200 and 6300 pumps.
[c]Tested in polyolefin containers.

Y-Site Injection Compatibility (1:1 Mixture)

			Paclitaxel				
Drug	*Mfr*	*Conc*	*Mfr*	*Conc*	*Remarks*	*Ref*	*C/I*
Ondansetron HCl	GL	0.03 and 0.3 mg/ml[a]	BR	0.3 mg/ml[a]	Visually compatible with no loss of either drug in 4 hr at 23 °C under fluorescent light	1741	**C**
	GL	0.03 and 0.3 mg/ml[a]	BR	1.2 mg/ml[a]	Visually compatible with no loss of either drug in 4 hr at 23 °C under fluorescent light	1741	**C**
Ondansetron HCl with ranitidine HCl	GL GL	0.3 mg/ml[a] 2 mg/ml[a]	BR	1.2 mg/ml[a]	Visually compatible with no loss of any drug by HPLC in 4 hr at 23 °C under fluorescent light	1741	**C**
Ranitidine HCl	GL	0.5 and 2 mg/ml[a]	BR	0.3 mg/ml[a]	Visually compatible with no loss of either drug in 4 hr at 23 °C under fluorescent light	1741	**C**
	GL	0.5 and 2 mg/ml[a]	BR	1.2 mg/ml[a]	Visually compatible with no loss of either drug in 4 hr at 23 °C under fluorescent light	1741	**C**

[a]*Tested in dextrose 5% in water.*

PHENOBARBITAL SODIUM
AHFS 28:12.04 and 28:24.04
Handbook on Injectable Drugs pp. 854–857

Drugs in Syringe Compatibility

			Phenobarbital sodium				
Drug (in syringe)	*Mfr*	*Amt*	*Mfr*	*Amt*	*Remarks*	*Ref*	*C/I*
Sufentanil citrate	JN	50 µg/ml	WY	60 mg/ml	Haze forms immediately and particles form in 24 hr at 23 °C	1711	**I**

Y-Site Injection Compatibility (1:1 Mixture)

			Phenobarbital sodium				
Drug	*Mfr*	*Conc*	*Mfr*	*Conc*	*Remarks*	*Ref*	*C/I*
Sufentanil citrate	JN	12.5 µg/ml[a]	WY	2 mg/ml[a]	Physically compatible with no change in measured turbidity or increase in particle content in 24 hr at 23 °C under fluorescent light	1711	**C**

[a]*Tested in dextrose 5% in water.*

PHENYTOIN SODIUM
AHFS 28:12.12
Handbook on Injectable Drugs pp. 861–867

Drugs in Syringe Compatibility

			Phenytoin sodium				
Drug (in syringe)	*Mfr*	*Amt*	*Mfr*	*Amt*	*Remarks*	*Ref*	*C/I*
Sufentanil citrate	JN	50 μg/ml	SO	50 mg/ml	Small crystals form immediately. Large crystals settle to bottom in 24 hr at 23 °C	1711	I

Y-Site Injection Compatibility (1:1 Mixture)

			Phenytoin sodium				
Drug	*Mfr*	*Conc*	*Mfr*	*Conc*	*Remarks*	*Ref*	*C/I*
Sufentanil citrate	JN	12.5 μg/ml[a]	ES	2 mg/ml[a]	Numerous tiny crystals form immediately and become larger over 24 hr at 23 °C under fluorescent light	1711	I

[a]*Tested in dextrose 5% in water.*

PIPERACILLIN SODIUM
AHFS 8:12.16
Handbook on Injectable Drugs pp. 870–875

Y-Site Injection Compatibility (1:1 Mixture)

			Piperacillin sodium				
Drug	*Mfr*	*Conc*	*Mfr*	*Conc*	*Remarks*	*Ref*	*C/I*
Teniposide	BR	0.1 mg/ml[a]	LE	40 mg/ml[a]	Physically compatible with no change in measured turbidity or increase in particle content in 4 hr at 23 °C under fluorescent light	1725	C

[a]*Tested in dextrose 5% in water.*

PLICAMYCIN
(MITHRAMYCIN)
AHFS 10:00
Handbook on Injectable Drugs pp. 881–883

Y-Site Injection Compatibility (1:1 Mixture)

			Plicamycin				
Drug	*Mfr*	*Conc*	*Mfr*	*Conc*	*Remarks*	*Ref*	*C/I*
Teniposide	BR	0.1 mg/ml[a]	MI	0.01 mg/ml[a]	Physically compatible with no change in measured turbidity or increase in particle content in 4 hr at 23 °C under fluorescent light	1725	C

[a]*Tested in dextrose 5% in water.*

POTASSIUM CHLORIDE
AHFS 40:12
Handbook on Injectable Drugs pp. 886–897

Y-Site Injection Compatibility (1:1 Mixture)

Drug	Mfr	Conc	Potassium chloride Mfr	Potassium chloride Conc	Remarks	Ref	C/I
Teniposide	BR	0.1 mg/ml[a]	AB	0.1 mEq/ml[a]	Physically compatible with no change in measured turbidity or increase in particle content in 4 hr at 23 °C under fluorescent light	1725	C

[a]*Tested in dextrose 5% in water.*

PROCAINAMIDE HCL
AHFS 24:04
Handbook on Injectable Drugs pp. 904–907

Additive Compatibility

Drug	Mfr	Conc/L	Procainamide HCl Mfr	Procainamide HCl Conc/L	Test Soln	Remarks	Ref	C/I
Flumazenil	RC	20 mg	ES	4 g	D5W[a]	Visually compatible with no flumazenil loss by HPLC in 24 hr at 23 °C under fluorescent light. Procainamide not tested	1710	C

[a]*Tested in PVC containers.*

PROCHLORPERAZINE EDISYLATE
AHFS 28:16.08 and 56.22
Handbook on Injectable Drugs pp. 910–916

Drugs in Syringe Compatibility

Drug (in syringe)	Mfr	Amt	Prochlorperazine edisylate Mfr	Prochlorperazine edisylate Amt	Remarks	Ref	C/I
Sufentanil citrate	JN	50 µg/ml	SCN	5 mg/ml	Physically compatible with no change in measured turbidity or increase in particle content in 24 hr at 23 °C under fluorescent light	1711	C

Y-Site Injection Compatibility (1:1 Mixture)

Drug	*Mfr*	*Conc*	*Mfr*	*Conc*	*Remarks*	*Ref*	*C/I*
			Prochlorperazine edisylate				
Sufentanil citrate	JN	12.5 μg/ml[a]	SCN	0.5 mg/ml[a]	Physically compatible with little change in measured turbidity or increase in particle content in 24 hr at 23 °C under fluorescent light	1711	C
Teniposide	BR	0.1 mg/ml[a]	SCN	0.5 mg/ml[a]	Physically compatible with no change in measured turbidity or increase in particle content in 4 hr at 23 °C under fluorescent light	1725	C

[a]*Tested in dextrose 5% in water.*

PROMETHAZINE HCL
AHFS 4:00 and 28:24.92
Handbook on Injectable Drugs pp. 920–927

Y-Site Injection Compatibility (1:1 Mixture)

Drug	*Mfr*	*Conc*	*Mfr*	*Conc*	*Remarks*	*Ref*	*C/I*
			Promethazine HCl				
Teniposide	BR	0.1 mg/ml[a]	WY	2 mg/ml[a]	Physically compatible with no change in measured turbidity or increase in particle content in 4 hr at 23 °C under fluorescent light	1725	C

[a]*Tested in dextrose 5% in water.*

RANITIDINE HCL
AHFS 56:40
Handbook on Injectable Drugs pp. 936–946

Additive Compatibility

Drug	*Mfr*	*Conc/L*	*Mfr*	*Conc/L*	*Test Soln*	*Remarks*	*Ref*	*C/I*
			Ranitidine HCl					
Fluconazole with ondansetron HCl	RR GL	2 g 100 mg	GL	500 mg	[a]	Visually compatible with no loss of any drug by HPLC in 4 hr	1730	C
Flumazenil	RC	20 mg	GL	300 mg	D5W[a]	Visually compatible with 3% flumazenil loss by HPLC in 24 hr at 23 °C under fluorescent light. Ranitidine not tested	1710	C

[a]*Tested in PVC containers.*

Y-Site Injection Compatibility (1:1 Mixture)

Drug	Mfr	Conc	Ranitidine HCl Mfr	Ranitidine HCl Conc	Remarks	Ref	C/I
Fluconazole	RR	2 mg/ml[a]	GL	0.5 and 2 mg/ml[b]	Visually compatible with no loss of either drug by HPLC in 4 hr	1730	C
Ondansetron HCl	GL	0.03, 0.1, 0.3 mg/ml[b]	GL	0.5 mg/ml[b]	Visually compatible with no loss of either drug by HPLC in 4 hr	1730	C
	GL	0.03, 0.1, 0.3 mg/ml[b]	GL	2 mg/ml[b]	Visually compatible with no loss of either drug by HPLC in 4 hr	1730	C
Ondansetron HCl with paclitaxel	GL BR	0.3 mg/ml[b] 1.2 mg/ml[b]	GL	2 mg/ml[b]	Visually compatible with no loss of any drug by HPLC in 4 hr at 23 °C under fluorescent light	1741	C
Paclitaxel	BR	0.3 mg/ml[b]	GL	0.5 and 2 mg/ml[b]	Visually compatible with no loss of either drug in 4 hr at 23 °C under fluorescent light	1741	C
	BR	1.2 mg/ml[b]	GL	0.5 and 2 mg/ml[b]	Visually compatible with no loss of either drug in 4 hr at 23 °C under fluorescent light	1741	C
Teniposide	BR	0.1 mg/ml[b]	GL	2 mg/ml[b]	Physically compatible with no change in measured turbidity or increase in particle content in 4 hr at 23 °C under fluorescent light	1725	C

[a]*Tested in sodium chloride 0.9%.*
[b]*Tested in dextrose 5% in water.*

SCOPOLAMINE HYDROBROMIDE (HYOSCINE HYDROBROMIDE) AHFS 12:08.08

Handbook on Injectable Drugs pp. 953–957

Drugs in Syringe Compatibility

Drug (in syringe)	Mfr	Amt	Scopolamine HBr Mfr	Scopolamine HBr Amt	Remarks	Ref	C/I
Sufentanil citrate	JN	50 μg/ml	LY	0.43 mg/ml	Physically compatible with no change in measured turbidity or increase in particle content in 24 hr at 23 °C under fluorescent light	1711	C

Y-Site Injection Compatibility (1:1 Mixture)

Drug	Mfr	Conc	Scopolamine HBr Mfr	Scopolamine HBr Conc	Remarks	Ref	C/I
Sufentanil citrate	JN	12.5 μg/ml[a]	LY	0.05 mg/ml[a]	Physically compatible with no change in measured turbidity or increase in particle content in 24 hr at 23 °C under fluorescent light	1711	C

[a]*Tested in dextrose 5% in water.*

SODIUM BICARBONATE
AHFS 40:08
Handbook on Injectable Drugs pp. 960–968

Drugs in Syringe Compatibility

			Sodium bicarbonate				
Drug (in syringe)	*Mfr*	*Amt*	*Mfr*	*Amt*	*Remarks*	*Ref*	*C/I*
Bupivacaine HCl	AST, WI	0.25, 0.5[a], 0.75%[a]; 20 ml	AB	4%, 0.05 to 0.6 ml	Precipitate forms in 1 to 2 min up to 2 hr at lowest amount of bicarbonate	1724	I
	BEL	0.5%[b], 20 ml		1.4%, 1.5 ml	Little or no loss of epinephrine by HPLC in 7 days at room temperature. Bupivacaine not tested	1743	C
	BEL	0.5%[b], 20 ml		4.2 and 8.4%, 1.5 ml	5 to 7% epinephrine loss by HPLC in 7 days at room temperature. Bupivacaine not tested	1743	C
Chloroprocaine HCl	AST	2 and 3%, 20 ml	AST	8.4%, 0.5 and 1 ml	Visually compatible for up to 5 hr at room temperature	1724	C
	AST	2 and 3%, 20 ml	AST	8.4%, 2 ml	Haze clarifies with gentle agitation	1724	?
	AST	2 and 3%, 20 ml	AB	4%, 1 and 2 ml	Visually compatible for up to 5 hr at room temperature	1724	C
	AST	2 and 3%, 20 ml	AB	4%, 4 ml	Haze clarifies with gentle agitation	1724	?
Etidocaine HCl[a]	AST	1 and 1.5%, 20 ml	AB	4%, 0.015 to 0.2 ml	Precipitate forms in 1 to 2 min to over 4 hr at lowest amount of bicarbonate	1724	I
Lidocaine HCl	ES	2%[c], 30 ml	AB	3 mEq/ 3 ml	11% lidocaine loss in 1 week and 22% loss in 2 weeks at 25 °C by GC. 28% epinephrine loss by HPLC in 1 week at 25 °C	1712	I
	ES	2%[c], 30 ml	AB	3 mEq/ 3 ml	6% lidocaine loss by GC in 4 weeks at 4 °C. 2% epinephrine loss in 1 week and 12% loss in 3 weeks at 4 °C by HPLC	1712	C
	AST	1%[c], 30 ml	LY	0.1 mEq/ml	25% epinephrine loss by HPLC in 1 week at room temperature. Lidocaine not tested	1713	I
		0.9%		0.088 mEq/ml	11% lidocaine loss by fluorescence polarization immunoassay in 7 days at room temperature	1723	C
	AST	1 and 1.5%[a], 20 ml	AST	8.4%, 2 ml	Visually compatible for up to 5 hr at room temperature	1724	C
	AST	2%[a], 20 ml	AST	8.4%, 2 ml	Haze clarifies with gentle agitation	1724	?
	AST	1 and 1.5%[a], 20 ml	AB	4%, 4 ml	Visually compatible for up to 5 hr at room temperature	1724	C
	AST	2%[a], 20 ml	AB	4%, 4 ml	Haze clarifies with gentle agitation	1724	?
	BEL	2%[d], 20 ml		1.4 and 8.4%, 1.5 ml	8% epinephrine loss by HPLC in 7 days at room temperature. Lidocaine not tested	1743	C
Mepivacaine HCl	AST, WI	1 and 1.5%, 20 ml	AST	8.4%; 0.5, 1, 2 ml	Precipitate forms within approximately 1 hr	1724	I
	AST, WI	1 and 1.5%, 20 ml	AB	4%; 1, 2, 4 ml	Precipitate forms within approximately 1 hr	1724	I

[a]Tested with and without epinephrine HCl 1:200,000 added.
[b]Tested with epinephrine HCl 1:200,000 added.
[c]Tested with epinephrine HCl 1:100,000 added.
[d]Tested with epinephrine HCl 1:80,000 added.

Y-Site Injection Compatibility (1:1 Mixture)

Drug	*Mfr*	*Conc*	**Sodium bicarbonate** *Mfr*	*Conc*	*Remarks*	*Ref*	*C/I*
Teniposide	BR	0.1 mg/ml[a]	AB	1 mEq/ml	Physically compatible with no change in measured turbidity or increase in particle content in 4 hr at 23 °C under fluorescent light	1725	C

[a]Tested in dextrose 5% in water.

STREPTOZOCIN
AHFS 10:00
Handbook on Injectable Drugs pp. 980–981

Y-Site Injection Compatibility (1:1 Mixture)

Drug	*Mfr*	*Conc*	**Streptozocin** *Mfr*	*Conc*	*Remarks*	*Ref*	*C/I*
Teniposide	BR	0.1 mg/ml[a]	UP	40 mg/ml[a]	Physically compatible with no change in measured turbidity or increase in particle content in 4 hr at 23 °C under fluorescent light	1725	C

[a]Tested in dextrose 5% in water.

TENIPOSIDE
AHFS 10:00
Handbook on Injectable Drugs pp. 984–986

Y-Site Injection Compatibility (1:1 Mixture)

Drug	*Mfr*	*Conc*	**Teniposide** *Mfr*	*Conc*	*Remarks*	*Ref*	*C/I*
Acyclovir sodium	BW	7 mg/ml[a]	BR	0.1 mg/ml[a]	Physically compatible with no change in measured turbidity or increase in particle content in 4 hr at 23 °C under fluorescent light	1725	C
Allopurinol	BW	3 mg/ml[a]	BR	0.1 mg/ml[a]	Physically compatible with no change in measured turbidity or increase in particle content in 4 hr at 23 °C under fluorescent light	1725	C
Amikacin sulfate	BR	5 mg/ml[a]	BR	0.1 mg/ml[a]	Physically compatible with no change in measured turbidity or increase in particle content in 4 hr at 23 °C under fluorescent light	1725	C
Aminophylline	AB	2.5 mg/ml[a]	BR	0.1 mg/ml[a]	Physically compatible with no change in measured turbidity or increase in particle content in 4 hr at 23 °C under fluorescent light	1725	C

Teniposide

Drug	*Mfr*	*Conc*	*Mfr*	*Conc*	*Remarks*	*Ref*	*C/I*
Amphotericin B	SQ	0.6 mg/ml[a]	BR	0.1 mg/ml[a]	Physically compatible with no change in measured turbidity or increase in particle content in 4 hr at 23 °C under fluorescent light	1725	C
Ampicillin sodium	WY	20 mg/ml[b]	BR	0.1 mg/ml[a]	Physically compatible with no change in measured turbidity or increase in particle content in 4 hr at 23 °C under fluorescent light	1725	C
Ampicillin sodium–sulbactam sodium	RR	20 + 10 mg/ml[b]	BR	0.1 mg/ml[a]	Physically compatible with no change in measured turbidity or increase in particle content in 4 hr at 23 °C under fluorescent light	1725	C
Aztreonam	SQ	40 mg/ml[a]	BR	0.1 mg/ml[a]	Physically compatible with no change in measured turbidity or increase in particle content in 4 hr at 23 °C under fluorescent light	1725	C
Bleomycin sulfate	BR	1 unit/ml[b]	BR	0.1 mg/ml[a]	Physically compatible with no change in measured turbidity or increase in particle content in 4 hr at 23 °C under fluorescent light	1725	C
Bumetanide	RC	0.04 mg/ml[a]	BR	0.1 mg/ml[a]	Physically compatible with no change in measured turbidity or increase in particle content in 4 hr at 23 °C under fluorescent light	1725	C
Buprenorphine HCl	RKC	0.04 mg/ml[a]	BR	0.1 mg/ml[a]	Physically compatible with no change in measured turbidity or increase in particle content in 4 hr at 23 °C under fluorescent light	1725	C
Butorphanol tartrate	BR	0.04 mg/ml[a]	BR	0.1 mg/ml[a]	Physically compatible with no change in measured turbidity or increase in particle content in 4 hr at 23 °C under fluorescent light	1725	C
Calcium gluconate	AMR	40 mg/ml[a]	BR	0.1 mg/ml[a]	Physically compatible with no change in measured turbidity or increase in particle content in 4 hr at 23 °C under fluorescent light	1725	C
Carboplatin	BR	5 mg/ml[a]	BR	0.1 mg/ml[a]	Physically compatible with no change in measured turbidity or increase in particle content in 4 hr at 23 °C under fluorescent light	1725	C
Carmustine	BR	1.5 mg/ml[a]	BR	0.1 mg/ml[a]	Physically compatible with no change in measured turbidity or increase in particle content in 4 hr at 23 °C under fluorescent light	1725	C

Teniposide

Drug	*Mfr*	*Conc*	*Mfr*	*Conc*	*Remarks*	*Ref*	*C/I*
Cefazolin sodium	MAR	20 mg/ml[a]	BR	0.1 mg/ml[a]	Physically compatible with no change in measured turbidity or increase in particle content in 4 hr at 23 °C under fluorescent light	1725	**C**
Cefonicid sodium	SKB	20 mg/ml[a]	BR	0.1 mg/ml[a]	Physically compatible with no change in measured turbidity or increase in particle content in 4 hr at 23 °C under fluorescent light	1725	**C**
Cefoperazone sodium	RR	40 mg/ml[a]	BR	0.1 mg/ml[a]	Physically compatible with no change in measured turbidity or increase in particle content in 4 hr at 23 °C under fluorescent light	1725	**C**
Cefotaxime sodium	HO	20 mg/ml[a]	BR	0.1 mg/ml[a]	Physically compatible with no change in measured turbidity or increase in particle content in 4 hr at 23 °C under fluorescent light	1725	**C**
Cefotetan disodium	STU	20 mg/ml[a]	BR	0.1 mg/ml[a]	Physically compatible with no change in measured turbidity or increase in particle content in 4 hr at 23 °C under fluorescent light	1725	**C**
Cefoxitin sodium	MSD	20 mg/ml[a]	BR	0.1 mg/ml[a]	Physically compatible with no change in measured turbidity or increase in particle content in 4 hr at 23 °C under fluorescent light	1725	**C**
Ceftazidime	LI	40 mg/ml[a]	BR	0.1 mg/ml[a]	Physically compatible with no change in measured turbidity or increase in particle content in 4 hr at 23 °C under fluorescent light	1725	**C**
Ceftizoxime sodium	FUJ	20 mg/ml[a]	BR	0.1 mg/ml[a]	Physically compatible with no change in measured turbidity or increase in particle content in 4 hr at 23 °C under fluorescent light	1725	**C**
Ceftriaxone sodium	RC	20 mg/ml[a]	BR	0.1 mg/ml[a]	Physically compatible with no change in measured turbidity or increase in particle content in 4 hr at 23 °C under fluorescent light	1725	**C**
Cefuroxime sodium	GL	20 mg/ml[a]	BR	0.1 mg/ml[a]	Physically compatible with no change in measured turbidity or increase in particle content in 4 hr at 23 °C under fluorescent light	1725	**C**
Chlorpromazine HCl	SCN	2 mg/ml[a]	BR	0.1 mg/ml[a]	Physically compatible with no change in measured turbidity or increase in particle content in 4 hr at 23 °C under fluorescent light	1725	**C**

Teniposide

Drug	*Mfr*	*Conc*	*Mfr*	*Conc*	*Remarks*	*Ref*	*C/I*
Cimetidine HCl	SKB	12 mg/ml[a]	BR	0.1 mg/ml[a]	Physically compatible with no change in measured turbidity or increase in particle content in 4 hr at 23 °C under fluorescent light	1725	C
Ciprofloxacin	MI	2 mg/ml[a]	BR	0.1 mg/ml[a]	Physically compatible with no change in measured turbidity or increase in particle content in 4 hr at 23 °C under fluorescent light	1725	C
Cisplatin	BR	1 mg/ml	BR	0.1 mg/ml[a]	Physically compatible with no change in measured turbidity or increase in particle content in 4 hr at 23 °C under fluorescent light	1725	C
Clindamycin phosphate	AST	10 mg/ml[a]	BR	0.1 mg/ml[a]	Physically compatible with no change in measured turbidity or increase in particle content in 4 hr at 23 °C under fluorescent light	1725	C
Cyclophosphamide	MJ	10 mg/ml[a]	BR	0.1 mg/ml[a]	Physically compatible with no change in measured turbidity or increase in particle content in 4 hr at 23 °C under fluorescent light	1725	C
Cytarabine	CET	50 mg/ml	BR	0.1 mg/ml[a]	Physically compatible with no change in measured turbidity or increase in particle content in 4 hr at 23 °C under fluorescent light	1725	C
Dacarbazine	MI	4 mg/ml[a]	BR	0.1 mg/ml[a]	Physically compatible with no change in measured turbidity or increase in particle content in 4 hr at 23 °C under fluorescent light	1725	C
Dactinomycin	MSD	0.01 mg/ml[a]	BR	0.1 mg/ml[a]	Physically compatible with no change in measured turbidity or increase in particle content in 4 hr at 23 °C under fluorescent light	1725	C
Daunorubicin HCl	WY	1 mg/ml[a]	BR	0.1 mg/ml[a]	Physically compatible with no change in measured turbidity or increase in particle content in 4 hr at 23 °C under fluorescent light	1725	C
Dexamethasone sodium phosphate	LY	1 mg/ml[a]	BR	0.1 mg/ml[a]	Physically compatible with no change in measured turbidity or increase in particle content in 4 hr at 23 °C under fluorescent light	1725	C
Diphenhydramine HCl	ES	2 mg/ml[a]	BR	0.1 mg/ml[a]	Physically compatible with no change in measured turbidity or increase in particle content in 4 hr at 23 °C under fluorescent light	1725	C

Teniposide

Drug	*Mfr*	*Conc*	*Mfr*	*Conc*	*Remarks*	*Ref*	*C/I*
Doxorubicin HCl	CET	2 mg/ml	BR	0.1 mg/ml[a]	Physically compatible with no change in measured turbidity or increase in particle content in 4 hr at 23 °C under fluorescent light	1725	**C**
Doxycycline hyclate	LY	1 mg/ml[a]	BR	0.1 mg/ml[a]	Physically compatible with no change in measured turbidity or increase in particle content in 4 hr at 23 °C under fluorescent light	1725	**C**
Droperidol	JN	0.4 mg/ml[a]	BR	0.1 mg/ml[a]	Physically compatible with no change in measured turbidity or increase in particle content in 4 hr at 23 °C under fluorescent light	1725	**C**
Enalaprilat	MSD	0.1 mg/ml[a]	BR	0.1 mg/ml[a]	Physically compatible with no change in measured turbidity or increase in particle content in 4 hr at 23 °C under fluorescent light	1725	**C**
Etoposide	BR	0.4 mg/ml[a]	BR	0.1 mg/ml[a]	Physically compatible with no change in measured turbidity or increase in particle content in 4 hr at 23 °C under fluorescent light	1725	**C**
Famotidine	MSD	2 mg/ml[a]	BR	0.1 mg/ml[a]	Physically compatible with no change in measured turbidity or increase in particle content in 4 hr at 23 °C under fluorescent light	1725	**C**
Floxuridine	RC	3 mg/ml[a]	BR	0.1 mg/ml[a]	Physically compatible with no change in measured turbidity or increase in particle content in 4 hr at 23 °C under fluorescent light	1725	**C**
Fluconazole	RR	2 mg/ml	BR	0.1 mg/ml[a]	Physically compatible with no change in measured turbidity or increase in particle content in 4 hr at 23 °C under fluorescent light	1725	**C**
Fludarabine phosphate	BX	1 mg/ml[a]	BR	0.1 mg/ml[a]	Physically compatible with no change in measured turbidity or increase in particle content in 4 hr at 23 °C under fluorescent light	1725	**C**
Fluorouracil	AD	16 mg/ml[a]	BR	0.1 mg/ml[a]	Physically compatible with no change in measured turbidity or increase in particle content in 4 hr at 23 °C under fluorescent light	1725	**C**
Furosemide	AB	3 mg/ml[a]	BR	0.1 mg/ml[a]	Physically compatible with no change in measured turbidity or increase in particle content in 4 hr at 23 °C under fluorescent light	1725	**C**

Teniposide

Drug	*Mfr*	*Conc*	*Mfr*	*Conc*	*Remarks*	*Ref*	*C/I*
Gallium nitrate	FUJ	0.4 mg/ml[a]	BR	0.1 mg/ml[a]	Physically compatible with no change in measured turbidity or increase in particle content in 4 hr at 23 °C under fluorescent light	1725	C
Ganciclovir sodium	SY	20 mg/ml[a]	BR	0.1 mg/ml[a]	Physically compatible with no change in measured turbidity or increase in particle content in 4 hr at 23 °C under fluorescent light	1725	C
Gentamicin sulfate	LY	5 mg/ml[a]	BR	0.1 mg/ml[a]	Physically compatible with no change in measured turbidity or increase in particle content in 4 hr at 23 °C under fluorescent light	1725	C
Haloperidol lactate	MN	0.2 mg/ml[a]	BR	0.1 mg/ml[a]	Physically compatible with no change in measured turbidity or increase in particle content in 4 hr at 23 °C under fluorescent light	1725	C
Heparin sodium	ES	100 units/ ml[a]	BR	0.1 mg/ml[a]	Physically compatible with no change in measured turbidity or increase in particle content in 4 hr at 23 °C under fluorescent light	1725	C
Hydrocortisone sodium phosphate	MSD	1 mg/ml[a]	BR	0.1 mg/ml[a]	Physically compatible with no change in measured turbidity or increase in particle content in 4 hr at 23 °C under fluorescent light	1725	C
Hydrocortisone sodium succinate	UP	1 mg/ml[a]	BR	0.1 mg/ml[a]	Physically compatible with no change in measured turbidity or increase in particle content in 4 hr at 23 °C under fluorescent light	1725	C
Hydromorphone HCl	KN	0.5 mg/ml[a]	BR	0.1 mg/ml[a]	Physically compatible with no change in measured turbidity or increase in particle content in 4 hr at 23 °C under fluorescent light	1725	C
Hydroxyzine HCl	WI	4 mg/ml[a]	BR	0.1 mg/ml[a]	Physically compatible with no change in measured turbidity or increase in particle content in 4 hr at 23 °C under fluorescent light	1725	C
Idarubicin HCl	AD	0.5 mg/ml[a]	BR	0.1 mg/ml[a]	Unacceptable increase in turbidity occurs immediately	1725	I
Ifosfamide	MJ	25 mg/ml[a]	BR	0.1 mg/ml[a]	Physically compatible with no change in measured turbidity or increase in particle content in 4 hr at 23 °C under fluorescent light	1725	C

Teniposide

Drug	*Mfr*	*Conc*	*Mfr*	*Conc*	*Remarks*	*Ref*	*C/I*
Imipenem–cilastatin sodium	MSD	10 mg/ml[b]	BR	0.1 mg/ml[a]	Physically compatible with no change in measured turbidity or increase in particle content in 4 hr at 23 °C under fluorescent light	1725	C
Leucovorin calcium	LE	2 mg/ml[a]	BR	0.1 mg/ml[a]	Physically compatible with no change in measured turbidity or increase in particle content in 4 hr at 23 °C under fluorescent light	1725	C
Lorazepam	WY	0.1 mg/ml[a]	BR	0.1 mg/ml[a]	Physically compatible with no change in measured turbidity or increase in particle content in 4 hr at 23 °C under fluorescent light	1725	C
Mannitol	WY	15%	BR	0.1 mg/ml[a]	Physically compatible with no change in measured turbidity or increase in particle content in 4 hr at 23 °C under fluorescent light	1725	C
Mechlorethamine HCl	MSD	1 mg/ml	BR	0.1 mg/ml[a]	Physically compatible with no change in measured turbidity or increase in particle content in 4 hr at 23 °C under fluorescent light	1725	C
Melphalan HCl	BW	0.1 mg/ml[a]	BR	0.1 mg/ml[a]	Physically compatible with no change in measured turbidity or increase in particle content in 4 hr at 23 °C under fluorescent light	1725	C
Meperidine HCl	WY	4 mg/ml[a]	BR	0.1 mg/ml[a]	Physically compatible with no change in measured turbidity or increase in particle content in 4 hr at 23 °C under fluorescent light	1725	C
Mesna	MJ	10 mg/ml[a]	BR	0.1 mg/ml[a]	Physically compatible with no change in measured turbidity or increase in particle content in 4 hr at 23 °C under fluorescent light	1725	C
Methotrexate sodium	LE	15 mg/ml[a]	BR	0.1 mg/ml[a]	Physically compatible with no change in measured turbidity or increase in particle content in 4 hr at 23 °C under fluorescent light	1725	C
Methylprednisolone sodium succinate	AB	5 mg/ml[a]	BR	0.1 mg/ml[a]	Physically compatible with no change in measured turbidity or increase in particle content in 4 hr at 23 °C under fluorescent light	1725	C
Metoclopramide HCl	ES	5 mg/ml	BR	0.1 mg/ml[a]	Physically compatible with no change in measured turbidity or increase in particle content in 4 hr at 23 °C under fluorescent light	1725	C

Teniposide

Drug	*Mfr*	*Conc*	*Mfr*	*Conc*	*Remarks*	*Ref*	*C/I*
Metronidazole	BA	5 mg/ml	BR	0.1 mg/ml[a]	Physically compatible with no change in measured turbidity or increase in particle content in 4 hr at 23 °C under fluorescent light	1725	**C**
Mezlocillin sodium	MI	40 mg/ml[a]	BR	0.1 mg/ml[a]	Physically compatible with no change in measured turbidity or increase in particle content in 4 hr at 23 °C under fluorescent light	1725	**C**
Miconazole	JN	3.5 mg/ml[a]	BR	0.1 mg/ml[a]	Physically compatible with no change in measured turbidity or increase in particle content in 4 hr at 23 °C under fluorescent light	1725	**C**
Minocycline HCl	LE	0.2 mg/ml[a]	BR	0.1 mg/ml[a]	Physically compatible with no change in measured turbidity or increase in particle content in 4 hr at 23 °C under fluorescent light	1725	**C**
Mitomycin	BR	0.5 mg/ml	BR	0.1 mg/ml[a]	Physically compatible with no change in measured turbidity or increase in particle content in 4 hr at 23 °C under fluorescent light	1725	**C**
Mitoxantrone HCl	LE	0.5 mg/ml[a]	BR	0.1 mg/ml[a]	Physically compatible with no change in measured turbidity or increase in particle content in 4 hr at 23 °C under fluorescent light	1725	**C**
Morphine sulfate	AST	1 mg/ml[a]	BR	0.1 mg/ml[a]	Physically compatible with no change in measured turbidity or increase in particle content in 4 hr at 23 °C under fluorescent light	1725	**C**
Nalbuphine HCl	DU	10 mg/ml	BR	0.1 mg/ml[a]	Physically compatible with no change in measured turbidity or increase in particle content in 4 hr at 23 °C under fluorescent light	1725	**C**
Netilmicin sulfate	SC	5 mg/ml[a]	BR	0.1 mg/ml[a]	Physically compatible with no change in measured turbidity or increase in particle content in 4 hr at 23 °C under fluorescent light	1725	**C**
Ondansetron HCl	GL	1 mg/ml[a]	BR	0.1 mg/ml[a]	Physically compatible with no change in measured turbidity or increase in particle content in 4 hr at 23 °C under fluorescent light	1725	**C**
Piperacillin sodium	LE	40 mg/ml[a]	BR	0.1 mg/ml[a]	Physically compatible with no change in measured turbidity or increase in particle content in 4 hr at 23 °C under fluorescent light	1725	**C**

Teniposide

Drug	*Mfr*	*Conc*	*Mfr*	*Conc*	*Remarks*	*Ref*	*C/I*
Plicamycin	MI	0.01 mg/ml[a]	BR	0.1 mg/ml[a]	Physically compatible with no change in measured turbidity or increase in particle content in 4 hr at 23 °C under fluorescent light	1725	**C**
Potassium chloride	AB	0.1 mEq/ml[a]	BR	0.1 mg/ml[a]	Physically compatible with no change in measured turbidity or increase in particle content in 4 hr at 23 °C under fluorescent light	1725	**C**
Prochlorperazine edisylate	SCN	0.5 mg/ml[a]	BR	0.1 mg/ml[a]	Physically compatible with no change in measured turbidity or increase in particle content in 4 hr at 23 °C under fluorescent light	1725	**C**
Promethazine HCl	WY	2 mg/ml[a]	BR	0.1 mg/ml[a]	Physically compatible with no change in measured turbidity or increase in particle content in 4 hr at 23 °C under fluorescent light	1725	**C**
Ranitidine HCl	GL	2 mg/ml[a]	BR	0.1 mg/ml[a]	Physically compatible with no change in measured turbidity or increase in particle content in 4 hr at 23 °C under fluorescent light	1725	**C**
Sodium bicarbonate	AB	1 mEq/ml	BR	0.1 mg/ml[a]	Physically compatible with no change in measured turbidity or increase in particle content in 4 hr at 23 °C under fluorescent light	1725	**C**
Streptozocin	UP	40 mg/ml[a]	BR	0.1 mg/ml[a]	Physically compatible with no change in measured turbidity or increase in particle content in 4 hr at 23 °C under fluorescent light	1725	**C**
Thiotepa	LE	1 mg/ml[a]	BR	0.1 mg/ml[a]	Physically compatible with no change in measured turbidity or increase in particle content in 4 hr at 23 °C under fluorescent light	1725	**C**
Ticarcillin disodium	BE	30 mg/ml[a]	BR	0.1 mg/ml[a]	Physically compatible with no change in measured turbidity or increase in particle content in 4 hr at 23 °C under fluorescent light	1725	**C**
Ticarcillin disodium–clavulanate potassium	SKB	31 mg/ml[a]	BR	0.1 mg/ml[a]	Physically compatible with no change in measured turbidity or increase in particle content in 4 hr at 23 °C under fluorescent light	1725	**C**
Tobramycin sulfate	LI	5 mg/ml[a]	BR	0.1 mg/ml[a]	Physically compatible with no change in measured turbidity or increase in particle content in 4 hr at 23 °C under fluorescent light	1725	**C**

Y-Site Injection Compatibility (1:1 Mixture) (Cont.)

Teniposide

Drug	*Mfr*	*Conc*	*Mfr*	*Conc*	*Remarks*	*Ref*	*C/I*
Trimethoprim–sulfamethoxazole	ES	0.8 + 4 mg/ml[a]	BR	0.1 mg/ml[a]	Physically compatible with no change in measured turbidity or increase in particle content in 4 hr at 23 °C under fluorescent light	1725	**C**
Vancomycin HCl	AB	10 mg/ml[a]	BR	0.1 mg/ml[a]	Physically compatible with no change in measured turbidity or increase in particle content in 4 hr at 23 °C under fluorescent light	1725	**C**
Vinblastine sulfate	LI	0.12 mg/ml[a]	BR	0.1 mg/ml[a]	Physically compatible with no change in measured turbidity or increase in particle content in 4 hr at 23 °C under fluorescent light	1725	**C**
Vincristine sulfate	LI	0.05 mg/ml[a]	BR	0.1 mg/ml[a]	Physically compatible with no change in measured turbidity or increase in particle content in 4 hr at 23 °C under fluorescent light	1725	**C**
Vinorelbine tartrate	BW	1 mg/ml[a]	BR	0.1 mg/ml[a]	Physically compatible with no change in measured turbidity or increase in particle content in 4 hr at 23 °C under fluorescent light	1725	**C**
Zidovudine	BW	4 mg/ml[a]	BR	0.1 mg/ml[a]	Physically compatible with no change in measured turbidity or increase in particle content in 4 hr at 23 °C under fluorescent light	1725	**C**

[a]*Tested in dextrose 5% in water.*
[b]*Tested in sodium chloride 0.9%.*

THEOPHYLLINE
AHFS 86:16

Handbook on Injectable Drugs pp. 987–989

Additive Compatibility

Theophylline

Drug	*Mfr*	*Conc/L*	*Mfr*	*Conc/L*	*Test Soln*	*Remarks*	*Ref*	*C/I*
Ceftriaxone sodium	RC	40 g	BA[a]	4 g		Yellow color forms immediately. 14% ceftriaxone loss and no theophylline loss by HPLC in 24 hr	1727	**I**

[a]*Tested in PVC containers.*

THIOTEPA
AHFS 10:00
Handbook on Injectable Drugs pp. 999–1000

Y-Site Injection Compatibility (1:1 Mixture)

			Thiotepa				
Drug	*Mfr*	*Conc*	*Mfr*	*Conc*	*Remarks*	*Ref*	*C/I*
Teniposide	BR	0.1 mg/ml[a]	LE	1 mg/ml[a]	Physically compatible with no change in measured turbidity or increase in particle content in 4 hr at 23 °C under fluorescent light	1725	C

[a]*Tested in dextrose 5% in water.*

TICARCILLIN DISODIUM
AHFS 8:12.16
Handbook on Injectable Drugs pp. 1000–1005

Y-Site Injection Compatibility (1:1 Mixture)

			Ticarcillin disodium				
Drug	*Mfr*	*Conc*	*Mfr*	*Conc*	*Remarks*	*Ref*	*C/I*
Teniposide	BR	0.1 mg/ml[a]	BE	30 mg/ml[a]	Physically compatible with no change in measured turbidity or increase in particle content in 4 hr at 23 °C under fluorescent light	1725	C

[a]*Tested in dextrose 5% in water.*

TICARCILLIN DISODIUM–CLAVULANATE POTASSIUM
AHFS 8:12.16
Handbook on Injectable Drugs pp. 1005–1007

Y-Site Injection Compatibility (1:1 Mixture)

			Ticarcillin disodium–clavulanate potassium				
Drug	*Mfr*	*Conc*	*Mfr*	*Conc*	*Remarks*	*Ref*	*C/I*
Teniposide	BR	0.1 mg/ml[a]	SKB	31 mg/ml[a]	Physically compatible with no change in measured turbidity or increase in particle content in 4 hr at 23 °C under fluorescent light	1725	C

[a]*Tested in dextrose 5% in water.*

TOBRAMYCIN SULFATE
AHFS 8:12.02
Handbook on Injectable Drugs pp. 1007–1016

Solution Compatibility

Tobramycin sulfate

Solution	*Mfr*	*Mfr*	*Conc/L*	*Remarks*	*Ref*	*C/I*
Dextrose 10% in water	SO	LI	60 mg/ 21.5 ml[a]	Visually compatible with little or no tobramycin loss by TDx in 30 days at 5 °C in the dark	1731	C
	SO	LI	60 mg/ 18.5 ml[a]	Visually compatible with little or no tobramycin loss by TDx in 30 days at 5 °C in the dark	1731	C
	SO	LI	120 mg/ 23 ml[a]	Visually compatible with little or no tobramycin loss by TDx in 30 days at 5 °C in the dark	1731	C
	SO	LI	120 mg/ 20 ml[a]	Visually compatible with little or no tobramycin loss by TDx in 30 days at 5 °C in the dark	1731	C

[a]*Tested in glass vials as a concentrate.*

Y-Site Injection Compatibility (1:1 Mixture)

Drug	*Mfr*	*Conc*	*Mfr*	*Conc*	*Remarks*	*Ref*	*C/I*
			Tobramycin sulfate				
Teniposide	BR	0.1 mg/ml[a]	LI	5 mg/ml[a]	Physically compatible with no change in measured turbidity or increase in particle content in 4 hr at 23 °C under fluorescent light	1725	C

[a]*Tested in dextrose 5% in water.*

TRIMETHOPRIM–SULFAMETHOXAZOLE (CO-TRIMOXAZOLE)
AHFS 8:40
Handbook on Injectable Drugs pp. 1023–1027

Y-Site Injection Compatibility (1:1 Mixture)

Drug	*Mfr*	*Conc*	*Mfr*	*Conc*	*Remarks*	*Ref*	*C/I*
			Trimethoprim + Sulfamethoxazole				
Teniposide	BR	0.1 mg/ml[a]	ES	0.8 + 4 mg/ml[a]	Physically compatible with no change in measured turbidity or increase in particle content in 4 hr at 23 °C under fluorescent light	1725	C

[a]*Tested in dextrose 5% in water.*

VANCOMYCIN HCL
AHFS 8:12.28
Handbook on Injectable Drugs pp. 1031–1038

Y-Site Injection Compatibility (1:1 Mixture)

			Vancomycin HCl				
Drug	*Mfr*	*Conc*	*Mfr*	*Conc*	*Remarks*	*Ref*	*C/I*
Cefotaxime sodium		100 mg/ml[a]		12.5, 25, 30, 50 mg/ml[a]	White precipitate forms immediately	1721	**I**
		100 mg/ml[a]		5 mg/ml[a]	No precipitate visually observed over 7 days at room temperature, but nonvisual incompatibility cannot be ruled out	1721	**?**
Teniposide	BR	0.1 mg/ml[b]	AB	10 mg/ml[b]	Physically compatible with no change in measured turbidity or increase in particle content in 4 hr at 23 °C under fluorescent light	1725	**C**

[a]*Tested in sterile water for injection.*
[b]*Tested in dextrose 5% in water.*

VINBLASTINE SULFATE
AHFS 10:00
Handbook on Injectable Drugs pp. 1047–1051

Y-Site Injection Compatibility (1:1 Mixture)

			Vinblastine sulfate				
Drug	*Mfr*	*Conc*	*Mfr*	*Conc*	*Remarks*	*Ref*	*C/I*
Teniposide	BR	0.1 mg/ml[a]	LI	0.12 mg/ml[a]	Physically compatible with no change in measured turbidity or increase in particle content in 4 hr at 23 °C under fluorescent light	1725	**C**

[a]*Tested in dextrose 5% in water.*

VINCRISTINE SULFATE
AHFS 10:00
Handbook on Injectable Drugs pp. 1051–1056

Y-Site Injection Compatibility (1:1 Mixture)

			Vincristine sulfate				
Drug	*Mfr*	*Conc*	*Mfr*	*Conc*	*Remarks*	*Ref*	*C/I*
Teniposide	BR	0.1 mg/ml[a]	LI	0.05 mg/ml[a]	Physically compatible with no change in measured turbidity or increase in particle content in 4 hr at 23 °C under fluorescent light	1725	**C**

[a]*Tested in dextrose 5% in water.*

ZIDOVUDINE
AHFS 8:18
Handbook on Injectable Drugs pp. 1058–1061

Y-Site Injection Compatibility (1:1 Mixture)

			Zidovudine				
Drug	*Mfr*	*Conc*	*Mfr*	*Conc*	*Remarks*	*Ref*	*C/I*
Teniposide	BR	0.1 mg/ml[a]	BW	4 mg/ml[a]	Physically compatible with no change in measured turbidity or increase in particle content in 4 hr at 23 °C under fluorescent light	1725	**C**

[a]*Tested in dextrose 5% in water.*

APPENDIX I: Parenteral Nutrition Solution Formulas

The following table summarizes the composition of the parenteral nutrition (TPN) solutions that are referenced throughout this Supplement. Each unique formula that was tested for stability and/or compatibility characteristics, alone or in combination with other drugs, is described and assigned a code number. These code numbers are used in the drug monographs to denote the TPN formulation being discussed (TPN #183, TPN #184, etc.). The TPN formulations are described as completely as possible from the original published sources.

		Concentration per Liter		
Component	Mfr	#183	#184	#185
Amino acids (Aminosyn II)	AB	1%	2.5%	5%
Dextrose	AB	10%	10%	25%
Calcium		9 mEq	4.4 mEq	5 mEq
Magnesium		5 mEq	5 mEq	5 mEq
Potassium		27 mEq	18 mEq	40 mEq
Sodium		24 mEq	38 mEq	42 mEq
Phosphorus		6 mM	9 mM	15 mM
Chloride		35 mEq	35 mEq	43 mEq
Acetate		22 mEq	25 mEq	38 mEq
Trace elements		1 ml	1 ml	1 ml

REFERENCES

1710. Olsen KM, Gurley BJ, Davis GA, et al.: Stability of flumazenil with selected drugs in 5% dextrose injection, *Am J Hosp Pharm 50*:1907–1912 (Sep) 1993.
1711. Trissel LA and Martinez JF: Sufentanil data on file, Pharmaceutical Analysis Laboratory, University of Texas, M. D. Anderson Cancer Center, Houston, Texas, February 1995.
1712. Larson PO, Ragi G, Swandby M, et al.: Stability of buffered lidocaine and epinephrine used for local anesthesia, *J Dermatol Surg Oncol 17*:411–414, 1991.
1713. Stewart JH, Cole GW, and Klein JA: Neutralized lidocaine with epinephrine for local anesthesia. *J Dermatol Surg Oncol 15*:1081–1083 (Oct) 1989.
1714. Nahata MC, Morosco RS, and Hipple TF: Stability of cimetidine hydrochloride and of clindamycin phosphate in water for injection stored in glass vials at two temperatures, *Am J Hosp Pharm 50*:2559–2561 (Dec) 1993.
1715. Zeisler J and Alagna C: Incompatibility of labetalol hydrochloride and furosemide, *Am J Hosp Pharm 50*:2521–2522 (Dec) 1993.
1716. Pfeifer RW and Hale KN: Precipitation of paclitaxel during infusion by pump, *Am J Hosp Pharm 50*:2518, 2521 (Dec) 1993.
1717. Hagan RL, Jacobs LF, Pimsler M, et al.: Stability of midazolam hydrochloride in 5% dextrose injection or 0.9% sodium chloride injection over 30 days, *Am J Hosp Pharm 50*:2379–2381 (Nov) 1993.
1718. Jones JW and Davis AT: Stability of bupivacaine hydrochloride in polypropylene syringes, *Am J Hosp Pharm 50*:2364–2365 (Nov) 1993.
1719. Vogt C, Skipper PM, and Ruggaber S: Compatibility of magnesium sulfate and morphine sulfate in 0.9% sodium chloride injection, *Am J Hosp Pharm 50*:2311 (Nov) 1993.
1720. Bailey LC, Tang KT, and Medwick T: Stability of ceftriaxone sodium in infusion-pump syringes, *Am J Hosp Pharm 50*:2092–2094 (Oct) 1993.
1721. Szof C and Walker PC: Incompatibility of cefotaxime sodium and vancomycin sulfate during Y-site administration. *Am J Hosp Pharm 50*:2054, 2057 (Oct) 1993.
1722. Jhee SS, Jeong EW, Chin A, et al.: Stability of ondansetron hydrochloride stored in a disposable, elastomeric infusion device at 4 °C, *Am J Hosp Pharm 50*:1918–1920 (Sep) 1993.
1723. Bartfield JM, Homer PJ, Ford DT, et al.: Buffered lidocaine as a local anesthetic: an investigation of shelf life, *Ann Emerg Med 21*:16–19 (Jan) 1992.
1724. Peterfreund RA, Datta A, and Ostheimer GW: pH adjustment of local anesthetic solutions with sodium bicarbonate: laboratory evaluation of alkalinization and precipitation, *Reg Aneth 14*:265–270 (Nov–Dec) 1989.
1725. Trissel LA and Martinez JF: Screening teniposide for Y-site physical incompatibilities, *Hosp Pharm 29*:1012–1014, 1017 (Nov) 1994.
1726. Woods K, Steinman W, Bruns L, et al.: Stability of foscarnet sodium in 0.9% sodium chloride injection, *Am J Hosp Pharm 51*:88–90 (Jan 1) 1994.
1727. Parrish MA, Bailey LC, and Medwick T: Stability of ceftriaxone sodium and aminophylline or theophylline in intravenous admixtures, *Am J Hosp Pharm 51*:92–94 (Jan 1) 1994.
1728. Lee MD, Hess MM, Boucher BA, et al.: Stability of amphotericin B in 5% dextrose injection stored at 4 or 25 °C for 120 hours, *Am J Hosp Pharm 51*:394–396 (Feb 1) 1994.
1729. Trissel LA and Martinez JF: Data on file, Pharmaceutical Analysis Laboratory, University of Texas, M. D. Anderson Cancer Center, Houston, Texas, November 1994.
1730. Pampilio FM, Fox JL, Inagaki K, et al.: Stability of ranitidine hydrochloride with ondansetron hydrochloride or fluconazole during simulated Y-site administration, *Am J Hosp Pharm 51*:391–394 (Feb 1) 1994.
1731. Wolff DJ, Kline SS, and Mauro LS: Stability of amikacin, gentamicin, or tobramycin in 10% dextrose injection, *Am J Hosp Pharm 51*:518–519 (Feb 15) 1994.
1732. Bosso JA, Prince RA, and Fox JL: Compatibility of ondansetron hydrochloride with fluconazole, ceftazidime, aztreonam, and cefazolin sodium under simulated Y-site conditions, *Am J Hosp Pharm 51*:389–391 (Feb 1) 1994.
1733. Stiles ML, Allen LV, Prince SJ, et al.: Stability of dexamethasone sodium phosphate, diphenhydramine hydrochloride, lorazepam, and metoclopramide hydrochloride in portable infusion-pump reservoirs, *Am J Hosp Pharm 51*:514–517 (Feb 15) 1994.
1734. Messerschmidt W: Kompatibilitat von ofloxacin mit ampicillin, *Krankenhauspharmazie 15*:337–340 (6) 1994.
1735. Messerschmidt W: Kompatibilitat von cefotaxim mit ofloxacin, *Pharmazie 136*:42–44 (Sep) 1991.
1736. Messerschmidt W: Kompatibilitat von cefuroxime mit metronidazol, *Krankenhauspharmazie 8*:45–47 (2) 1987.
1737. Messerschmidt W: Kompatibilitat von cefotiam mit metronidazol, *Krankenhauspharmazie 7*:263–265 (6) 1986.
1738. Messerschmidt W: Pharmazeutische kompatibilitat der kombination cefotiam und ampicillin, *Krankenhauspharmazie 13*:98–100 (3) 1992.
1739. Belliveau PP, Nightingale CH, and Quintiliani R: Stability of aztreonam and ampicillin sodium–sulbactam sodium in 0.9% sodium chloride injection, *Am J Hosp Pharm 51*:901–904 (Apr 1) 1994.
1740. Frase GL and Riker RR: Visual compatibility of haloperidol lactate with injectable solutions, *Am J Hosp Pharm 51*:905–906 (Apr 1) 1994.
1741. Burm JP, Jhee SS, Chin A, et al.: Stability of paclitaxel with ondansetron hydrochloride or ranitidine hydrochloride during simulated Y-site administration. *Am J Hosp Pharm 51*:1201–1204 (May 1) 1994.
1742. Mulye NV, Turco SJ, and Speaker TJ: Stability of ganciclovir sodium in an infusion-pump syringe, *Am J Hosp Pharm 51*:1348–1349 (May 15) 1994.
1743. Bonhomme L, Benhamou D, Comoy E, et al.: Stability of adrenaline pH-adjusted solutions of local anaesthetics, *J Pharm Biomed Anal 9*:497–499 (6) 1991.
1744. Johnson CE, Jacobson PA, and Chan E: Stability of ganciclovir sodium and amino acids in parenteral nutrient solutions, *Am J Hosp Pharm 51*:503–508 (Feb 15) 1994.
1745. Trissel LA, Xu Q, Martinez JF, et al.: Compatibility and stability of ondansetron hydrochloride with morphine sulfate and with hydromorphone hydrochloride in 0.9% sodium chloride injection at 4, 22, and 32 °C, *Am J Hosp Pharm 51*:2138–2142 (Sep 1) 1994.
1746. Xu Q, Trissel LA, and Martinez JF: Stability of paclitaxel in 5% dextrose injection or 0.9% sodium chloride injection at 4, 22, or 32 °C, *Am J Hosp Pharm 51*:3058–3060 (Dec 15) 1994.

ASHP'S *INFUSION TECHNOLOGY MANUAL & VIDEOTAPE:*

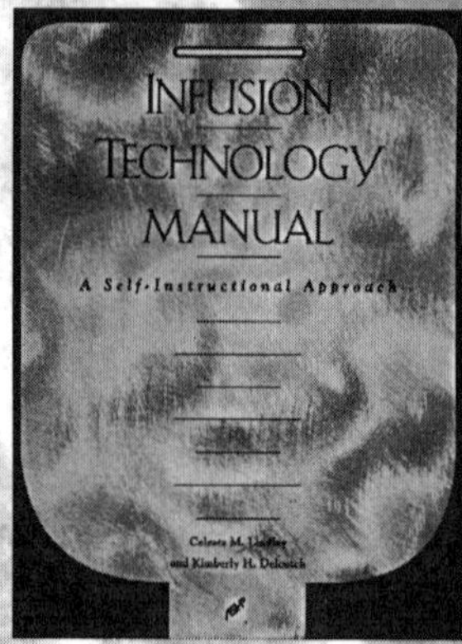

Learn the basics of infusion technology with ASHP's *Infusion Technology Manual & Videotape: A Self-Instructional Approach* By Celeste M. Lindley & Kimberly H. Deloatch

This manual teaches pharmacists about various aspects of infusion technology. Chapters cover the following:

- History and overview of parenteral therapy
- Routes of parenteral therapy and therapeutic indications
- Complications of intravenous therapy
- Basic concepts of fluid dynamics
- Vascular access devices
- Infusion control devices
- And more!

Each chapter includes learning objectives, a summary, and self-assessment questions. The manual also includes standards for parenteral drug therapy, references, and a list of infusion control device manufacturers.

This book is an excellent training tool for pharmacy personnel and students with limited infusion-related practice experience. You can order the manual separately or the manual with the companion videotape.

The videotape part of this package has been contributed by Abbott Hospital Products Division.

American Society of Health-System Pharmacists®

ORDER FORM

- **MANUAL ONLY, Please send me _____ copies of**
  Infusion Technology Manual: A Self-Instructional Approach (P413) at:
  $50 ASHP Members (please provide ASHP member ID#) **$63** Full Price
- **MANUAL & VIDEOTAPE, Please send me _____ copies of**
  Infusion Technology Manual and Videotape: A Self-Instructional Approach (P415) at:
  $175 ASHP Members (please provide ASHP member ID#) **$219** Full Price

(Note: Canadian orders add 25% surcharge for GST and brokerage fees.)

NAME: ____________________

ADDRESS: ____________________
(include name of institution, if applicable)
____

CITY: __________ **STATE:** __________ **ZIP:** __________

DAY PHONE: ( ) __________ **ASHP MEMBER ID #:** __________
(must include to receive member price)

- Enclosed is my **check** for $ _______ made payable to ASHP and drawn on a U.S. bank.
- Enclosed is our **U.S. purchase order #** __________ for $ __________
  (Please issue an invoice and add postage and handling)
- **Charge** $ _______ to my:
  VISA   American Express   MasterCard   Discover

Account #: ____________________ Exp. date: __________
month/ year

Cardholder's Signature: ____________________

Mail to: ASHP Customer Service, 7272 Wisconsin Avenue, Bethesda, MD 20814
Phone to: 301-657-4383 **FAX to:** 1-800-665-ASHP

FAX and phone orders, please have your credit card or purchase order number ready.

All ASHP products come with a 30-day money-back guarantee. Payments to ASHP are not deductible as charitable contributions for federal income tax purposes. However, they may be deductible under other provisions of the Internal Revenue Code.

©1995 American Society of Health-System Pharmacists

Save time. Avoid mistakes. Answer injectable drug questions with confidence.

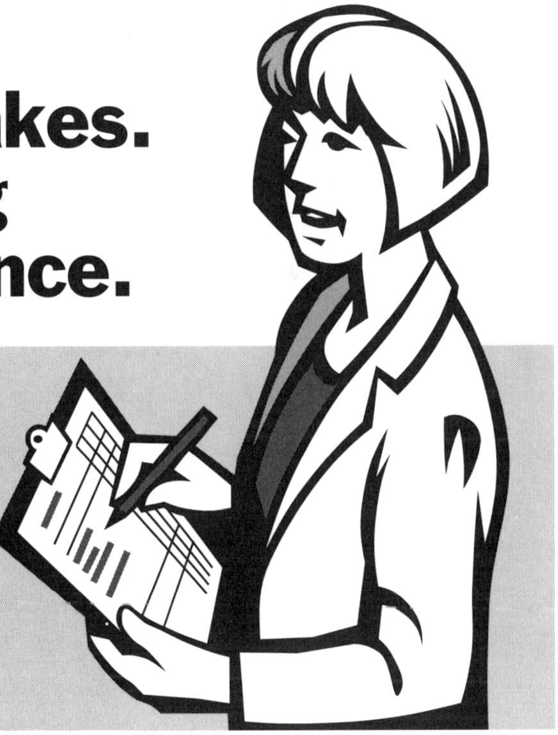

Carry the
Pocket Guide to Injectable Drugs

Companion to
Handbook on Injectable Drugs,
8th Edition by Lawrence A. Trissel

Are these two drugs compatible in solution?
What is the recommended concentration?
How is the drug diluted?
Can the drug be given an IV push?
How long is the drug stable in solution?

As the drug therapy expert, you're frequently called upon to answer questions like these. Or, you may be required to join patient rounds and provide on-the-spot advice. Don't be caught off-guard— carry the concise but thorough *Pocket Guide to Injectable Drugs!*

- Provides monographs on 116 of the most commonly-prescribed injectable drugs.
- Includes hard-to-find compatibility information in an easy-to-use, tabular format.
- Answers questions on products, preparation, dosage, administration, compatibility, stability, and pharmacology.
- Portable size is there when you need it — no matter where you are or what time of day it is!

Stay current with the new edition, which includes dozens of updates from previous editions, as well as brand new drug monographs including:

- Atracurium besylate
- Carboplatin
- Diltiazem HCl
- Filgrastim
- Gallium nitrate
- Idarubicin HCl
- Paclitaxel
- Piperacillin sodium-tazobactam sodium
- Ticarcillin disodium-clavulanate potassium

Carry the **Pocket Guide to Injectable Drugs**—*because patients are depending on you!*

ASHP

ASHP Guarantee:
We are so sure our products will meet your needs, we provide a 30-day, money-back guarantee. If you are not satisfied with any ASHP product, simply return it within 30 days of purchase for a full refund!

Method of Payment
☐ Check payable to ASHP and drawn on a U.S. bank.
☐ U.S. purchase order #______________ please issue an invoice and add postage & handling.
☐ Charge my: ☐ VISA ☐ MC ☐ Disc. ☐ AmEx
Account # ______ Exp. Date ______ *(mo./yr.)*
Signature ______

Bulk quantity and university discounts available.

Payments to ASHP are not deductible as charitable contributions for federal income tax purposes. However, they may be deductible under other provisions of the Internal Revenue Code.

©1994 American Society of Health-System Pharmacists

Mail: ASHP Customer Service
7272 Wisconsin Ave., Bethesda, MD 20814

Fax: 301/657-1251 **Phone:** 301/657-4383
Please have your credit card or purchase order # ready.

Name ______ Daytime Phone ______
Position/Title ______ Organization ______
Address ______
City ______ State ______ Zip ______

To receive ASHP member discount, please provide your **ASHP Member ID#**______
☐ Please send me a complete ASHP Products and Services Catalog.

Product	Order Code	ASHP Member	ASHP Student	Full Price	Quantity	Total Price
Pocket Guide to Injectable Drugs	**P445**	**$25**	**$19**	**$41**		
Handbook on Injectable Drugs, 8th Edition	**P423**	**$100**	**$75**	**$135**		

Canadian GST Fees

Order Total	Add	Order Total	Add	Order Total	Add
$0.01-$60	35%	$61-$80	30%	$81-$120	25%
$121-$260	20%	$261-$1,000	15%	$1,001	10%

Canadian orders add appropriate surcharge (see table) to cover GST and brokerage fees.

International orders, please add $10 per product.

Total Order ______